"*Breathe In Calm* is a wise, kind, and beautiful offering. This book provides practica[l] [...] [li]ve better with anxiety for a lifet[ime]

—Bob Stahl, P[hD]

Based Stress Reduction [...]

Date: 1/27/22

615.82 WEG
Wegesin, Domonick,
Breathe in calm : yogic
breathing & mindfulness

ck

"*Breathe In Calm* is a lifesaver for anyone that has ever experienced anxiety. The simple yet powerful tools and practices are explained in a clear, practical, and easy-to-follow manner. The book reflects Domonick Wegesin's years of experience helping people navigate anxiety through his deep mastery of science, yoga, and mindfulness."

> —**Ashley Sharp,** longtime yoga and meditation
> teacher, author of *Mindfulness for Beginners*,
> and founder of Refuge at Pudding Creek—
> a retreat center in Northern California

"*Breathe In Calm* is a timely and significant book; a vital antidote to the increased anxiety in our lives. Wegesin lives and writes with the integrity garnered from experience. The mindfulness toolbox of compassionate practices cultivates the healing power of the breath, a 'self-psychology' that is always effective and available to us. I look forward to enthusiastically recommending this book to both colleagues and clients!"

—**Preston Parsons, LCSW**, psychotherapist,
consultant, and mindfulness practitioner

"*Breathe In Calm* is a breath of fresh air for anyone who experiences anxiety on any level, which means all of us. Wegesin's evidence-based approach is both accessible and affirming. Combining cutting-edge neuroscience with the potent sharing of various students/clients who have successfully integrated these practices into their lives, this guide is as groundbreaking as it is grounding. Equal parts wisdom and wit, this book is bound to change your life."

—**Ken Breniman, LCSW**, somatic psychotherapist,
certified yoga therapist, thanatologist,
and psychedelic and plant medicine
integration specialist

breathe in calm

in calm

yogic breathing &
mindfulness tools *for*
instant anxiety relief

DOMONICK WEGESIN, PHD

New Harbinger Publications, Inc.

Publisher's Note

Distributed in Canada by Raincoast Books

NEW HARBINGER PUBLICATIONS is a registered trademark of New Harbinger Publications, Inc.

Copyright © 2021 by Domonick Wegesin
New Harbinger Publications, Inc.
5674 Shattuck Avenue
Oakland, CA 94609
www.newharbinger.com

Cover design by Sara Christain; Interior design by Amy Shoup and Michele Waters-Kermes; Acquired by Georgia Kolias; Edited by Jennifer Eastman

"Peace Is This Moment Without Judgment," Leaves from Moon Mountain: Poems and Reflections by Dorothy Hunt. Collage art by Rashani Réa. San Francisco: Moon Mountain Sangha Publishing, 2015, p. 132. Reprinted with permission.

Library of Congress Cataloging-in-Publication Data

Names: Wegesin, Domonick, author.
Title: Breathe in calm : yogic breathing and mindfulness tools for instantanxiety relief / Domonick Wegesin, PhD.
Identifiers: LCCN 2021026549 | ISBN 9781684038817 (trade paperback)
Subjects: LCSH: Yoga--Therapeutic use. | Anxiety disorders--Alternative treatment. | Breathing exercises--Therapeutic use.
Classification: LCC RM727.Y64 W44 2021 | DDC 615.8/24--dc23
LC record available at https://lccn.loc.gov/2021026549

Printed in the United States of America

23   22   21

10   9   8   7   6   5   4   3   2   1   First Printing

I dedicate this book to all of my students who, over the years, have taught me so much about applying these mindful tools to real life. Thank you for your vulnerability, courage, and willingness to turn toward your anxiety with more compassion. Without your inspiration, I would not have written this book.

I also dedicate this offering to you, the reader. May these tools be of service to you in exploring and understanding the pain caused by your anxiety. May these words help you find relief from that pain.

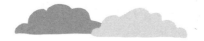

Contents

Introduction: Anxiety and the Tools to Relieve It

Not long after moving to New York City, I enjoyed a delightful Sunday bike ride along the Hudson River north of the city. On my way back to Manhattan, I was racing down a long hill, feeling elated by the beautiful day, when an oncoming car took a quick left-hand turn and crossed unexpectedly in front of me. I had only seconds to slam on my brakes before colliding with the car. I remember flying upward and then waking up in the middle of the road some time later, unable to move. The vehicle had fled the scene. I suppose that the driver didn't want to be held accountable for my injuries after cutting in front of me when I had the right of way.

I was lucky. My now-broken helmet took the brunt of the impact, but my bones remained intact. What was troubling, however, was the automatic reaction my body started having to traffic after the accident. New York pedestrians are not great observers of the don't walk sign, and I jaywalked with the best of them. However, after the accident, my body would seize up any time I needed to cross a street, even when the walk signal assured my right of way. My breath would tighten, my heart would race, my muscles would clench, and my brain would paint gruesome scenarios of getting smashed by buses or slammed by taxis. I was a nervous wreck, even walking a few blocks to the subway.

The physiological changes that I experienced are part of the body's fight-or-flight response. Your brain evolved to set off internal alarms at the approach of predators or the expectation of danger, which tell you to fight, flee, or freeze. Ideally, after the threat has passed, the fight-or-flight system switches off, and you calm down. This process is hard-wired through evolution and is critical for your survival, so it's not something you can just uninstall.

Unfortunately, your fight-or-flight system can get stuck in a state of arousal, even when nothing threatening is happening. Your brain perceives that you are in danger when, in fact, you are safe. There are many reasons why this can happen: accidents, surgeries, chronic stress, bullying, emotional neglect, or any other kind of trauma. It could be a combination of things. Most anxious folks cannot pinpoint exactly why they are anxious. That's okay. There's a simpler way.

Instead of getting distracted by asking *why* you are anxious, *Breathe In Calm* will teach you to focus on *what*.

- What are your anxious symptoms?

- What are your triggers?

- What are your reactions to anxiety?

- What can you do to calm your anxiety?

- What will help you shift your relationship to anxiety so that it bothers you less?

We'll learn and use a small but powerful set of tools—Observer, Breathing, Grounding, Acceptance, Choice, Story, and Kindness. Each of these tools will take its place in an overall strategy to transform your own personal relationship with your anxiety.

First, before you try to calm your anxiety, you have to realize that you're feeling anxious. This may sound elementary, but anxiety often is happening without your being fully aware of it. You may habitually hold tension in your shoulders, bite your nails, avoid eye contact, or feel restless without fully realizing it. Your mind is good at distracting you from anxious symptoms to avoid dwelling in the discomfort associated with them. However, in this mindful approach, you will turn your attention toward your anxiety in order to work with it more skillfully. Don't worry if you're not great at noticing all of your anxious habits yet, because the Observer Tool will improve your ability to notice anxious symptoms as soon as they appear.

Your anxiety tends to snowball. It may start with a single worrisome thought, then build as other related anxious thoughts pop into your mind. Within a short time, your anxiety ramps up to the point where you start to feel overwhelmed. You're not alone! The trick is to catch the cycle of anxiety early, as it's easier to unplug from anxiety when it's only a whisper. Conversely, it's much harder to calm anxiety once it has snowballed into a panic. With these mindfulness tools, you will get better at detecting the early hints of anxiety to help you disarm an anxious cycle before it becomes a problem.

Once you become aware of anxiety, then you will learn to calm your body's fight-or-flight response using the Breathing, Grounding, and Acceptance Tools. With these tools, you'll soon become a pro at relaxing yourself quickly and easily. These calming tools are critical, because when you are responding from fear, you automatically react based on your survival needs. Your brain tells you to flee, fight, or freeze. These responses are, by evolutionary design, quick and unconscious. This is referred to as "amygdala hijacking."

The amygdala is your brain's watchdog, always monitoring the environment for potential threats. When the amygdala sounds the alarm, your attention gets hyperfocused on what is upsetting you. Your memory recalls anything relevant to that upset. Stress hormones flood your body and further increase your anxious arousal. The slower, more evolved parts of your brain take a back seat, making it hard for you to think clearly. Your ability to generate ideas, reason, or solve problems is impaired. As psychologists say, "When you are stressed, you regress." You've surely noticed how anxiety can muck up your thinking.

Once you've started to calm the siren of your fear brain, you can then use the Choice Tool to respond to upsetting interactions. Choice involves managing how you're investing your attention so that you don't waste time and energy stuck in worries and ruminations. And perhaps more importantly, choice involves determining your attitude toward anxiety. If you hate your anxiety, you empower it to bother you more. But if you accept your anxious experience, it loses its power over you. Shifting your attitude will decrease the pain that anxiety produces.

Finally, the Kindness Tool helps you to relate to yourself and others with greater friendliness, especially when you're anxious. Self-criticism is a hallmark of anxiety. When you're anxious, you're more likely to judge yourself harshly. As you can imagine, self-criticism only adds to your anxiety. Replacing criticism with kindness is the remedy, as it's hard for your brain to be kind and anxious at the same time. Choosing kindness provides an excellent antidote for anxiety.

Now, before we begin, I want to highlight the experiential nature of this book. The primary teacher will be your own first-hand experience using the tools I describe. To help you, each chapter includes practice sections. Some are formal meditations, in which you set aside time to cultivate mindfulness. Some are informal practices, in which you incorporate the mindful techniques you are learning into your everyday life. Others are reflection exercises, in which you journal about your relationship to anxiety. All are important.

To help you become comfortable with these meditations and exercises, there are materials available for download on this book's website, including audio recordings of meditations and photographs to illustrate yoga poses. These can be found at http://www.newharbinger.com/48817.

Most anxious people have an efficiency expert installed in their brains, which makes them want to rush through a book in order to finish it as quickly as possible. *Ding!* Another item checked off of your to-do list. That impulse will prod you to skip the practice exercises. Please don't succumb to that temptation. Instead, acknowledge the impulse to rush ahead, then choose to do the exercises anyway. This gives you a chance to learn how to use your Choice Tool to override automatic impulses so that you can develop better self-care. You have to take time for yourself. If you engage in the exercises, I'm confident the tools in this book will help you to feel less anxious and more whole. Let's get started!

The Observer Tool

One of my students, Ann, came for a consultation with complaints of fatigue and worry. She was going through a divorce and found herself worrying about her financial stability, her job prospects after being a stay-at-home mom, her kids missing their dad, and her prospects of feeling good enough to want to date again. She also wondered about what her friends would think of her divorce, worrying about which ones might side with her husband and gossip behind her back. Even though she was exhausted, she just couldn't get a good night's sleep. Her worries spun into the small hours of the night. If she did fall asleep, she'd wake up in the middle of the night with a mind whirling in fear. She was frazzled, yet still felt antsy and keyed up.

Ann's symptoms probably sound familiar. Many of us are juggling the activities of daily life while simultaneously trying to manage our anxiety. Researchers have found that a worrying brain consumes up to twenty times the amount of energy it uses when it's not worrying. Unsurprisingly, people with anxiety often feel burned out.

What may be initially disappointing to hear is that freeing yourself from anxiety doesn't involve eliminating anxiety entirely. It's a hardwired part of the human brain—we're stuck with it. You can learn to be less anxious and experience fewer symptoms, but even then, you'll still have anxious moments. So instead of eliminating anxiety, you are going to change your relationship to it. When you're not trying to avoid it, control it, or distract yourself from it, it bothers you less. In brief, you will learn how to navigate anxiety more mindfully.

To begin your mindful journey, we'll start with the Observer Tool, which helps you notice when, where, and how anxiety shows up. Without awareness, anxiety keeps chugging along habitually, often without you being fully aware of its presence. Only by noticing that you are having an anxious moment are you able to do something about it.

1. Mindfulness

Mindfulness originates from a 2,500-year-old Buddhist meditation tradition. It was popularized in the United States by Dr. Jon Kabat-Zinn, who developed the mindfulness-based stress reduction program (MBSR). Mindfulness involves how you use your attention to affect your experience.

William James, one of the founding fathers of American psychology, wrote, "My experience is what I agree to attend to."[1] Or, in the parlance of the modern life coach, "energy flows where attention goes." Learning to manage how you invest your attention can have an enormous impact on how you experience your life.

Think of your mind as a stage and your attention as a spotlight that shines on just one actor at a time. In any given moment, many things are vying for your attention. Some of them are internal, like an ache in your back, a feeling of loneliness, or a memory of a childhood friend. Some of them are external, like a ringing phone or the sight of your dog greeting you at the door when you get home. But in any given moment, your mind's spotlight focuses on just one out of those thousands of things. What you *notice* at that moment forms your *experience* of that moment.

Although paying attention is essential for learning and understanding, our educational system doesn't provide training on how to develop your attentional skills, other than our teachers badgering us to "Pay attention!" William James wrote, "The faculty of voluntarily bringing back a wandering attention, over and over again, is the very root of judgment, character, and will… An education which should improve this faculty would be the education par excellence."[2]

Mindfulness provides the exact type of attention training that James touted. It helps you choose where you focus your mind. Your attention is your most valuable resource. Think about it; everyone wants to get your attention: family, friends, work, social media. Online advertisers use ethically questionable techniques to capture your attention, leading you to waste time on things that aren't important. Mindfulness helps you become a better chooser of how you invest your limited attentional resources. To be mindful, you'll learn to pay attention in three ways:

- purposefully
- non-judgmentally
- non-elaboratively

Purposefully

Usually, your mind is operating on automatic pilot. For example, one minute you are busy at work, and the next, you are rehashing an upsetting conversation you had with a friend. You didn't choose to drum up that conversation; it just popped into your head on its own. Automatic pilot is the mind's default mode. Mindful attention is different in that you purposefully choose to put your mind on a specific thought, emotion, sense, or action.

Non-Judgmentally

Anxious minds are judgmental minds. You're quick to rate your experiences: good or bad, pleasant or unpleasant, right or wrong. These verdicts arrive so speedily that they can seem to be part of the experience itself. However, when you stop to consider it, you see that the judgment of the experience is different than the experience itself. For example, if your friend is telling you about a guy she just met, and your mind is thinking, *OMG, he sounds like a real loony,* you are no longer hearing your friend, you are judging her choices.

Judgments often distort reality to fit your expectations of how you think the world should be, how other people should be, or how you should be. The distortions can be so powerful that you perceive what you *expect* rather than what is actually there. The poet Anaïs Nin cleverly reflected these perceptual distortions by saying, "We don't see the world as it is, we see the world as we are."[3]

There's a fun baby shower game called "name that poop" that demonstrates how the mind distorts reality. In the game, various foods are served inside a diaper. When seeing melted chocolate, your mind perceives the brown in the diaper as poop, and you experience disgust. Your expectation of what *should* be in a diaper (poop) overrides your perception of what *is* in the diaper (chocolate). Even when your rational brain says, "I know it's just chocolate," it can still be hard to override your disgust. Someone watching you eat chocolate out of a diaper would also experience disgust.

Mindfulness helps you notice these distortions so that you can begin to see the world more objectively. The distortions often amplify your anxiety as your fear brain paints trouble where none objectively exists. You imagine people criticizing you or imagine that you'll ruin an upcoming project. You might get overwhelmed by events that do not go the way you expect. By letting go of the judgment of how you think life should be, you can better go with the flow of how life actually is. From that objective perspective, you'll feel less bothered by unpleasant experiences, which will make it easier for you to accept life's natural ups and downs.

Non-Elaboratively

Similarly to the way that your mind automatically judges your experiences, it also tends to elaborate on them. For example, imagine seeing a girl riding her bike on the sidewalk. Your mind embellishes the sight by recalling a bike-riding memory from your childhood or from when you taught your daughter to ride. You can get easily lost in a whole cascade of related and unrelated thoughts without consciously noticing them. Though this type of self-referential elaboration is normal, it can distract you from what is happening in the here and now.

When your mind has the habit of being anxious, these elaborations are often tinged with negativity. They often produce more anxious thoughts, which propel you into a spiral of anxiety. With mindfulness, you develop the ability to pay attention without getting lost in elaborations. When you notice elaborations, you choose to refocus on what is happening in the here and now.

2. Shine Your Attention's Spotlight

Okay, now that you have a definition of mindfulness, let's start to learn *how* to be mindful. Let me return to the analogy of your mind as a stage. Wherever your attentional spotlight shines makes up your experience of that moment. If you are attending to washing dishes, then dishwashing is your experience of that moment. However, if you are going through the motions of dishwashing, but your mind is worrying about how your son is getting along with his friends, then your experience of that moment is worry. What is important to realize is that you can control the spotlight. You can choose to shift focus from worry back to dishwashing.

Shifting the spotlight is easy, but it happens only when you are awake to that moment. Most of the time, the spotlight is driven automatically, by your habits. In those moments, you aren't choosing where your attention goes, it just goes where it has habitually gone before. For example, if you have the habit of worrying, the mind easily switches back to worry. If you're a planner, then the spotlight is drawn to planning.

To use your Observer Tool, you have to step into the role of the spotlight operator and choose what to focus on. In the theater, the spotlight operator is not there to critique the performers, add lines to the performance, or create a ruckus that distracts from the actors. The spotlight operator just focuses the attention of the audience. When you use your Observer Tool, you learn to witness what is happening without attaching or identifying with what you notice, judging what you observe, or running from what is present. You just watch.

PRACTICE

Let's try taking your Observer Tool out for a little spin. First, notice something you see, and note to yourself, "I see _____." Then notice something you hear, and note, "I hear _____." In the same way, notice things you smell, taste, and feel. Now, notice any emotions you are experiencing. Finally, observe what thoughts are on your mind.

As you observed these different things, did you judge them? For example, did you think, *I like that sound*? Did you elaborate on any of the experiences? For example, if you saw a letter on your desk, did you remember that you forgot to send your mother a birthday card last week? For now, notice how quickly and automatically these judgments and elaborations happen. But also notice how you can observe the judgments and elaborations. For example, *I'm judging the sound of the traffic as pleasant. Judgment is here.* Or *I'm thinking about why I am feeling sad. Elaborative thinking is here.* No matter what your experience is, you can observe it objectively with your Observer Tool.

3. Observing Your Anxiety

Now you're ready to hone your Observer Tool to see exactly how anxiety shows up in your life. You may already feel overly familiar with your anxiety and cringe at the idea of examining it further. But remember that if you are going to do anything about your anxious symptoms, you first need to become aware of them. So let's break down common symptoms into four categories: physical, emotional, mental, and behavioral.

Physical Sphere	Emotional Sphere
muscle tension	uneasiness
sleep disturbance	distractibility
elevated pulse	feeling overwhelmed
disturbed breathing	panic
frequent fatigue	irritability

Thought Sphere	Behavioral Sphere
worry	avoidance
racing thoughts	restlessness
obsession	erratic movements
apprehension	impulsive behavior
catastrophizing	rapid speech

PRACTICE

Though you may relate to many of these examples, I'd like you to create your own personal list. Make a note on your phone or in your journal and add items whenever you notice them throughout the day. Keep track of repetitions of your symptoms with a running tally next to each symptom. This will help you understand the most frequent ways anxiety shows up for you.

One important caveat when doing this awareness practice is that by paying more attention to your anxiety, it's likely that you will notice anxious symptoms more frequently. You may misinterpret the increase in frequency of *noticing* anxiety as an increase in anxiety itself. Keep in mind that much of your anxiety usually goes on under the radar of your conscious awareness. Your Observer Tool is not adding to your anxiety; it is drawing back the curtain to reveal the pervasiveness of the anxiety that already exists. So if you do find that you are noticing more anxiety, it's actually a sign that you are using the Observer Tool. Keep up the good work!

Granted, it's easy to get frustrated when you notice how often you experience anxiety. To reduce that frustration, it helps to note your symptoms with an objective tone, rather than a judgmental one. Think of yourself as a scientist observing a guinea pig (but in this case, you are both the scientist and the guinea pig). The scientist wants to report what the guinea pig does without judging it as good or bad, right or wrong. Everything you notice is information that will help you understand how, when, and where your anxiety manifests. You are already on your way to coping better.

4. Noting

Noting involves silently naming what you notice. You acknowledge where your attention has landed in that moment. It makes explicit the things your mind does automatically. You might note to yourself, *Listening to this podcast, Smelling coffee, Worrying about my kids,* or *Tying my shoes.* It is best to keep a light touch when you note things. Try not to elaborate on what you notice; simply acknowledge what's happening in that moment.

My student Rachel, who experienced panic attacks and was diagnosed with generalized anxiety disorder, described how noting helped her manage her symptoms: "Once I became familiar with the symptoms of my anxiety, I could notice when they were coming. Noting allowed me to recognize what was happening without getting overwhelmed by my anxiety. Simply naming what I am feeling is tremendously helpful. I find that from the place of the noter, I can feel my anxiety and let it pass without it spiraling into a full-blown panic attack, which is what used to happen before I learned these tools."

Noting reflects what psychologists call "distancing." It adds a little distance between you and what you are experiencing. Distancing can create enough wiggle room between you and your problems so that you feel less bothered them. When you feel less bothered, it's easier to make smarter choices about how to deal with the problem at hand.

It's especially helpful to use an objective tone when noting. The way you typically talk about your emotions can make them seem more permanent than they actually are. For example, when you say, "I'm anxious," it almost sounds like a declaration of who you are, rather than a description of a passing emotional condition. Though it may sound awkward at first, try saying, "Anxiety is here."

You may also notice how your self-referential statements often are tinged with judgment. For example, "Oh crap, my anxious indigestion is back." You can hear your disdain for the symptom, even if it is just in your tone of voice. The "oh crap" relays judgment about the indigestion, and the "my" makes it seem like a permanent personal trait. Both the judgment and personalization keep you stuck in those conditions longer. Being non-judgmental and objective helps you stay centered in yourself as you let your experiences come and go.

PRACTICE

Developing the habit of using more objective language takes time. To practice, try rephrasing subjective sentences to be more objective. For example, instead of "Ugh, I'm so worried about his friends not liking me," say "Worrying about his friends not liking me is here." Rephrase the following in a journal.

- Darn it, I'm biting my nails again.

- OMG, this awful jaw clenching is driving me crazy.

- I hate feeling so antsy.

5. Peaceful Pause

Most anxious folks tend to be perpetually on the go. From the moment you get up, go through your morning bathroom routine, make breakfast, and commute to work, you are running from one thing to the next. Even when your body is not on the move, your mind races with upcoming plans or rehashes past events. A mind that is constantly swept into the future or sucked back into the past is not well equipped to deal with what's on your plate right now.

The Peaceful Pause trains you to slow down enough to step out of the incessant *doing* in order to shift into *being* with the present moment. Since our culture prioritizes productivity, we are trained to believe that our value corresponds to how busy we are. Accordingly, pausing even for a moment may make you feel like you are wasting time or being lazy. Pausing and observing is especially challenging for anxious people, whose brains are hyperaroused and less able to inhibit automatic thoughts. Try to notice your reaction to pausing without judging it as wrong, even if it feels uncomfortable. If pausing frustrates you, note, "Frustration is here."

PRACTICE

Stop what you are doing and ask, "What's here now?" Do you notice thoughts, emotions, sights, sounds, smells, sensations, or habits? Remember that you don't need to fix anything, improve anything, or avoid anything. Simply observe what is here.

Probably the biggest challenge in mindfulness is remembering to be mindful. These tools don't do you any good unless you put them to use. So, to help build mindfulness into your routine, I recommend setting a Peaceful Pause alarm on your phone to remind you to pause at regular intervals (try hourly). You might feel overly distracted by your phone already, and you might resist using it to help you here. But in this case, it's not leading you into mindless doom scrolling; it's reminding you to take a Peaceful Pause. Let your technology help you. If you'd rather establish a non-digital reminder, consider attaching your Peaceful Pauses to an activity you frequently do, like drinking water or sitting down. Each time you start that activity, inject a Peaceful Pause. In this way, you start to integrate mindfulness into your everyday life.

6. The Anxiety Snowball

One of my mindfulness students, Carol, described an incident at work where she forgot to set up a digital projector for a group meeting. Though it only took her a few minutes to set it up once the meeting started, she felt embarrassed for making everyone wait. During the meeting, her memory slip cascaded into an avalanche of anxious ruminations about what her colleagues thought of her. This snowballed to more catastrophic thoughts: *I'm such a failure. Everyone here thinks I'm stupid. I'm going to get fired.* Within minutes, her initial worry about forgetting the projector became a storm of anxious self-talk that left her feeling miserable all day.

You have undoubtedly experienced snowballing, where one little mishap cascades into drama that is disproportionate to the mishap. A key element of this training is to catch anxiety before it snowballs out of control. It is easier to calm yourself when your symptoms are just a whisper, rather than waiting until you are near panic before intervening. The take-home message is that as soon as you notice anxious symptoms, use your calming tools (the Grounding and Breathing Tools, which are coming soon) to settle yourself.

Your body registers fear before your mind picks up on it as a thought. Thus, body-based symptoms are some of your best early detectors of anxiety. However, our thinking culture trains us to be more tuned into thoughts than into our bodies. To become a better listener to your body's cues, you'll next learn the Body Scan.

7. Body Scan Meditation

The Body Scan is your first formal mindfulness meditation to build awareness. As the title implies, you will scan through different parts of your body and feel whatever sensations you notice. Some sensations you'll feel on the surface, like the coolness of the air on your skin or the touch of fabric from your shirt. Some sensations are deeper, like feeling your pulse. Focus on whatever sensations you feel. When your mind wanders to something else, gently but firmly return your attention to the sensations. Like most mindfulness practices, understanding how to do the Body Scan is pretty easy. Actually getting your mind to cooperate is where it gets to be more challenging. Be patient as you begin to train your brain to be more mindful. The Body Scan provides four important benefits in working with anxiety.

First, it helps build your Observer Tool by training your attention. While focusing on body sensations, your mind wanders away to think of something else. You note the distraction and then redirect your attention back to the body. This improves your ability to put your attention where you want it to be.

Second, the Body Scan increases your sensitivity to how your body communicates with you through sensations, changes in breath rate, and muscle tension. With greater awareness of your body, you will be able to detect subtle changes in your physiological state associated with anxiety.

Third, the Body Scan builds your Acceptance and Kindness Tools. The anxious mind is hypercritical: *I'm so stupid* or *I'm too old*. You apply that same criticism to your body, *I'm not strong enough, I hate my thighs,* or *I feel gross*. Needing your body to be somehow different than it is in order for you to be happy contributes to your anxiety. With acceptance, you develop a kinder relationship to your body and begin to loosen up on the self-criticism that keeps you feeling bad. In the Body Scan, you practice letting your body be just as it is. When you accept yourself more, it's easier to be more accepting of others. This simple meditation becomes a vehicle for improving social justice, reducing bias and criticism against people who differ from you.

Finally, the Body Scan creates a greater sense of well-being by naturally relaxing your body. Anxiety makes your muscles tense up. Picture your body cowering in fear: scrunched shoulders, ducked head, tightened jaw, caved spine, clenched butt, and gripped stomach. Chronic anxiety creates a more temperate version of that response, with your body continuously girding itself against potential harm.

The state of your body influences the state of your mind, and vice versa. For example, chronic tension in your shoulders sends a message to the brain that protection is needed; this keeps the mind on alert for trouble. Conversely, relaxed shoulders send a message that the environment is safe, and the mind can relax. Accordingly, you can reduce your mental anxiety by reducing your body tension. Think of how you feel after a hot bath, massage, or yoga class. The Body Scan likewise releases physical tension to help you feel more at peace.

PRACTICE

There are many ways to do a Body Scan. You can use the guided meditation on the book's website (http://www.newharbinger. com/48817—audio accessory 1: Body Scan Meditation) or the instructions below.

Process. For this meditation, find a comfortable position lying down. Scan through your body and feel the sensations that you notice. Focus your attention on the sensations in each body part for one minute, then move on. This is just a suggested order: (1) belly, (2) left hand, (3) left arm, (4) left and right shoulders, (5) right arm, (6) right hand, (7) ten toes, (8) both feet, (9) both legs, (10) pelvis, (11) back, (12) face, (13) nose.

Acceptance. Your mind will label some sensations pleasant and others unpleasant. Try to release judging the sensations. Instead, cultivate the attitude, *Okay, this is just how things are right now.* If you try to fight off unpleasant thoughts, emotions, or body sensations, your struggle will create more unpleasantness. If you allow your experience to be as it is, then you will create more peace.

Mind-wandering. Just as the salivary glands secrete saliva, the mind secretes thoughts. You will be distracted while you meditate. Whatever arises—thoughts, emotions, recognition of sounds—just note the distraction and return your attention to feeling your body. It can be frustrating noticing how often your mind wanders. Simply note—*Frustration is happening*—and return to your body.

Congratulate yourself when you manage to refocus on your body. By framing those mindful reawakenings as victories, you will release some feel-good dopamine into your brain. Getting upset over mind-wandering is an example of your mind creating a problem where no problem exists. Don't indulge your drama-maker; the world has enough drama in store for you already.

Some people become worried when they can't feel parts of their body, imaging that something must be wrong. It's very unlikely that anything is wrong. It's just that we don't spend much time feeling our bodies, so our brains don't prioritize that ability. With practice, you will become more sensitive to subtle sensations. It can be like tuning in to a distant radio station. Initially, you hear only a crackle of a sound, but as you hone your attention and adjust the dial, the signal becomes clearer.

Your mind likes to tell stories about your body. For instance, focusing on your knees may cue a memory, *Oh, I remember the time I twisted my knee hiking.* However, thinking about sensations is different than feeling sensations. If you notice stories about what you are feeling, note to yourself, *Thinking,* and return to feeling.

Regardless of what happens during the Body Scan, if you are constantly distracted, fall asleep, or feel antsy, just try to observe and accept your experience. Some days will be easier than others. The effects of the training will differ across sessions. Let go of judging your ability as good or bad and the meditation as a success or a failure. Simply *practicing it* is a success, no matter how it turns out.

SUMMARY OF THE OBSERVER TOOL

Anxiety is a habit that runs on automatic pilot, often without your being aware of it. Only by first noticing that you are having an anxious moment can you then do something about it. You have begun to use your Observer Tool to become aware of your experience in the present moment and to familiarize yourself with the various ways in which anxiety expresses itself. Noting your symptoms objectively helps you distance yourself from them. As you continue to practice this, you will notice that the symptoms bother you less.

Now that you've learned how to notice when anxiety shows up, let's begin to explore how to calm yourself when you feel anxious.

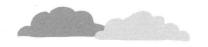

The Breathing Tool

Every fall, one of my students, Ashley, dreads having to give a presentation to the parents of her incoming elementary school students. Leading up to the presentation, she feels her chest tighten and her breath shorten. Sometimes it feels like she can't breathe at all, and that makes her even more anxious. She worries that her nervousness will make a bad impression on the parents.

Ashley's breathing difficulties are common among people with anxiety. Anxious breaths are fast and constrained to the upper lungs.[4] Scientists have shown that fast, shallow breathing triggers mechanisms within the amygdala, your brain's threat monitor, similar to those triggered by anxiety. In fact, the activity of your amygdala tends to sync up with your breath rate.[5] When shallow breathing becomes a habit, the fight-or-flight system is continually revving up your anxiety. This chronic stress has several harmful side effects:

- upset digestion,[6]

- sleep disturbances,[7]

- reduction in attention and memory,[8] and

- decreased immune function, making you more susceptible to illness.[9]

One of the frustrations about working with anxiety is the feeling that it is out of your control. You start to become anxious about being anxious. That is, you worry that anxiety will take over at an inopportune time and embarrass you or interfere with your ability to function. Learning to reduce your anxiety with breathing gives you a sense of control, trusting that you can calm yourself any time you need to. That's why the Breathing Tool is so important, because when you believe in your ability to self-calm, you will feel less victimized by anxiety and worry less about it showing up.

Not only is breathing effective, but it also acts faster than anxiety medication, providing more immediate relief from your anxious symptoms. It often works even when talk therapy doesn't, because it affects the amygdala, which is such an ancient part of your brain that it doesn't respond well to thought-based approaches. As an added bonus, breathing costs nothing and doesn't come with all the side effects of pharmaceutical remedies. (However, most users do become dependent on breathing, and withdrawal is inevitably fatal.)

If you're wondering why short, shallow breathing activates your fight-or-flight response, it's because anxious breathing is associated with the most primal threat detector, smell. All animals use their senses to detect threats. Humans have evolved to rely more on vision, but other animals still rely more on smell. You've probably seen a dog sniff the air when it checks out a new place. Those short, rapid sniffs stimulate the dog's fight-or-flight system, helping it be hypervigilant, scanning the area for anything amiss.

If you smell smoke, your amygdala rings the alarm and sends a message telling your nose to sniff more to suss out where the smoke is coming from. So the sniffing breath has become connected with your fight-or-flight system. Even though anxious breathers aren't sniffing for scents, the short, shallow breaths resemble sniffing enough to trigger the brain's alarm.

In contrast, slow breathing calms the fight-or-flight response to reduce your anxiety.[10] My student Ashley learned to use controlled breathing to calm herself before giving her presentation.

This year was my most successful presentation, in large part due to mindfulness and controlled breathing. Every time I felt a wave of nervousness I noted, "Nervousness is here," and practiced controlled breathing. It calmed me down. I did this several times in the hours leading up to the presentation and experienced a wave of calm each time. Once the presentation began, I felt more at ease than I ever had before. When I felt nervous during the presentation, I would take a slow breath, and it calmed me. Since I was calmer, I was more confident talking with parents and answering their questions. In the past, I would drive home feeling embarrassed. This year I drove home feeling proud.

Controlled breathing works for everyday anxieties but can also reduce symptoms of anxiety and depression in patients with generalized anxiety disorder.[11] In fact, controlled breathing can be effective even when you don't get relief from anxiety medications.[12] Controlled breathing also works for people with severe anxiety, like panic and PTSD.[13]

8. Rapid Breathing and Panic

Phoebe was having a difficult month. Her mother had just passed away after a fight with breast cancer. She was behind at work from having taken time off to care for her mom in hospice. She also hadn't had time to exercise. One afternoon at the grocery, she started to have difficulties breathing. The lights in the store seemed to get brighter, and she felt as if people were crowding in around her. She then felt weak in the knees and thought she was about to die. Her breath got faster and more labored. Finally, she collapsed. Later Phoebe reported that she thought she must have had a heart attack, but at the hospital her heart checked out fine. Instead, her doctor diagnosed a panic attack.

So how does rapid breathing lead to a full-blown panic attack? The quick answer is hyperventilation. Let me explain. Your body is always balancing the oxygen it takes in and the carbon dioxide it sends out. Too much oxygen makes you feel agitated and jumpy. Too much carbon dioxide makes you feel sluggish and tired.

When people with anxiety take short breaths, it sometimes feels like they're not getting enough oxygen, so they compensate by taking faster breaths. However, the feeling of not getting enough breath is actually caused by getting too much oxygen, not too little. When you breathe these rapid, shallow breaths, you expel too much carbon dioxide. Overall, breathing faster adds too much oxygen and worsens the feelings of agitation and breathlessness.

Anxious breathing kicks your nervous system into overdrive and leads to hyperventilation. Have you ever experienced symptoms like lightheadedness, chest pain, leg weakness, or rapid heartbeat? This could be caused by anxious breathing. Many people, like Phoebe, report feelings of impending doom, which naturally cause more anxiety and disturbed breathing. You spiral in a vicious upward cycle in which anxious thoughts evoke anxious breathing, which stir feelings of panic, which causes faster breathing, which can lead to a full-blown panic attack. People with a history of panic develop the habit of overbreathing to try to avoid the feeling of breathlessness their panic attacks produce.

The traditional trick of breathing into a paper bag actually works to calm you down, because inhaling the carbon dioxide you just exhaled rebalances the oxygen–carbon dioxide ratio. Luckily, deep yogic breathing also rebalances the breath, so you don't have to always walk around with a paper bag handy.

9. Slow Breathing

Given that your fear brain tends to override your higher brain when you get upset, the logical thing to do when you notice anxious symptoms is first to calm your fear brain. One of the fastest ways to do so is with slow, deep breathing. Then once your higher brain is back in charge, you can respond more skillfully to the problem at hand.

Sometimes when people try to slow their breath, they get too full of breath while inhaling or run out of breath too early while exhaling. Overfilling the lungs can make your cardiovascular system work overtime, which can create more anxiety. So you need to slow not only the *timing* of your breath but also the *rate* of your breath. For this, we'll use a yogic breath called *ujjayi* [pronounced "oodge-eye"] breathing. This breath creates a sound like the ocean heard inside a seashell. *Ujjayi* breathing will help you develop greater breath awareness and control.

PRACTICE

To begin, imagine breathing on the mirror in your bathroom to fog it up: open your mouth and exhale. It makes a *hhhhhhaa* sound. Feel the light friction in the back of your throat. That is what helps you control the rate at which the breath passes through the airway. Now try with your lips closed. It's quieter, but you can still hear it. Finally, experiment with making the ocean sound as you inhale. This may feel funny at first, because it is new to your vocal cords. Don't worry—it gets easier with practice. As a rule, yogic breathing is done through the nose for both inhales and exhales. However, if you are congested, it's fine to breathe through your mouth.

Practice the *ujjayi* breath for two minutes. Listen to the ocean sound it makes as you breathe. Try to make the inhales and exhales sound alike. Notice how you feel after just two minutes of slow, controlled breathing.

10. Deep Belly Breathing

Great! Now that you have learned to slow your breath, let's explore how to deepen it. Your lungs are covered with the nerves of your rest and digest system, which helps calm you after an upset. These are especially abundant in the lower lobes of your lungs; that's how deep belly breathing can have such a powerfully calming effect. To practice, allow your belly to gently expand like a balloon as you inhale. Let it relax as you exhale.

Side note: Given our culture's obsession with toned abs, you may be reluctant to let your belly widen for yogic breathing. Don't worry, deep breathing is not going to make you fat or make your belly hang out. It will help you calm down, so you worry less about your weight and appearance. Bonus!

Since anxious people have excess muscle tension and tend to over-strive, it is important to keep your exhales easy. If you forcefully push the breath out, then this practice can have the unintended effect of making you tenser.

As visual creatures, we typically focus on what we can see. So when asked to breathe more deeply, most people push their front ribs forward. Try that with your next inhale. However, when you push your front ribs forward notice how the back of your body tenses, your back muscles contract, and your shoulder blades pull closer to each other. This is not helpful. You actually have more space to breathe in your back ribs than your front ribs. Anecdotally, you may have heard of COVID patients being placed belly-down in their hospital beds—this is done so that they can take advantage of back breathing.

To use your full lung capacity, picture a balloon inflating and deflating, expanding and contracting evenly all the way around, and let your torso mimic the balloon, expanding in all directions—front, back, and sides. Then let your belly and ribs gently settle back toward midline as you exhale. Again, don't strive. Keep it feeling easy.

PRACTICE

You may follow the guided meditation for belly breathing on the book's website (http://www.newharbinger.com/48817—audio accessory 2: Belly Breathing) or use the instructions here.

Find a comfortable seated position. If you are sitting in a chair, scooch forward a little so your back is not touching the seat back. Place your palms on your lower belly. As you inhale, feel the belly expand into your palms. Take five front belly breaths.

Next, shift your hands to touch your side belly, between the hip and ribs. Can you feel the side belly expand as you inhale? Take five more breaths into your side belly.

Then touch your lower back and feel five back breaths expanding there.

Finally, release your hands and imagine an inner tube wrapped around you at belly level. As you inhale, expand the inner tube in in all directions. Feel the sensations of expansion as you inhale. As you exhale, let the inner tube deflate.

Learning belly breathing can be challenging at first, due to the tenacity of your current breathing habits, which have developed over your lifetime. These habits can change, but it takes time and practice.

One nice perk of breathing practice is that you can do it anywhere. For example, many of us get anxious when we have to wait. So next time you are waiting for a friend, instead of jumping on your phone, practice breathing. It'll make waiting more relaxing, and you won't be so angry at your friend for being late. Mindful win!

11. Relaxation Breathing

Now you know how to breathe slowly and deeply to calm your anxiety. This is already a tremendous asset, which I encourage you to practice frequently. The more you use it, the easier and more effective it becomes.

However, sometimes you might need a stronger dose of calming. Introducing Relaxation Breathing. In this breathing technique, you will change the ratio of your breath to induce states of deep peace and well-being.

Breathing is the second most important tool in your toolbox, following the Observer Tool, and Relaxation Breathing is one of the best breathing techniques for calming your system. First, you become aware that you are experiencing anxiety. Then you calm your fight-or-flight response with Relaxation Breathing.

PRACTICE

You may practice on your own, using the instructions below, or follow the guided practice on the book's website (http://www.newharbinger.com/48817—audio accessory 3: Relaxation Breathing).

For Relaxation Breathing, you will exhale longer than you inhale. For example, you might inhale for three seconds and then exhale for six seconds. Feel welcome to adjust the timing so that it's comfortable for you. Applying the *ujjayi* technique will help you slow and smooth your exhale. If you start to feel short of breath or challenged, don't exhale quite so long.

The relaxation effect can be enhanced further by adding a short pause after you exhale. For example, inhale three seconds, exhale six seconds, and then pause, with your lungs empty, for three seconds. Again, if this pattern feels challenging, reduce the duration of the exhale or the pause to find something more manageable.

To begin, try a few rounds of Relaxation Breathing *without* the empty pause, breathing in three seconds and then breathing out six seconds. If that feels comfortable, try adding the pause after you exhale: inhale three seconds, exhale six seconds, and pause empty three seconds. Practice for two minutes, then take a break to notice how you feel.

During the day, as soon as you detect anxious symptoms, apply Relaxation Breathing. With repeated practice, you'll become an expert at calming yourself quickly and easily.

12. Bee's Breath

Across time and cultures, singing has been used as a mood lifter. The Bee's Breath applies humming to clear the mind of worries and to alleviate insomnia. While these instructions apply specifically to the Bee's Breath, you can benefit from any type of humming, like humming your favorite songs.

PRACTICE

Find a comfortable seated position. Take a full belly breath in, then hum your exhales, making a long *mmmm* sound. As you hum, focus your attention on the vibration the humming creates around your nose and mouth. To help you focus, close your eyes and plug your ears. Practice for two minutes. Once you are done humming, feel the leftover vibrations still buzzing in your face. Imagine these tingly sensations moving into other parts of your body. Allow your body to be soft and receptive, so that the vibration can flow into different body parts. After a couple of minutes, note the effects of the practice. Do you feel calmer? Is your mind clearer?

13. Awareness of Breath

Even when you don't control it, focusing on your breath can be calming. Attending to your breath brings your attention immediately back to the here and now and pulls you out of anxious ruminations. When you concentrate on managing what's happening right now, you usually realize that in this moment you are okay, and that this moment is manageable. Looking into the future with an anxious mind creates unneeded upset.

Practicing Awareness of Breath further bolsters your ability to pay attention, which is critical to improving your Observer Tool. You'll get better at noticing what you're focusing on, and switching to focus on what you choose, rather than letting your automatic fear brain take the reins and orient you toward worries and upsets.

After having practiced controlled breathing, it may be hard to release control of your breath. If so, simply note, *Controlling*, and try to let the body just breathe by itself. Anxious people have a tendency to be controlling. We feel that keeping other people and things in check will reduce the likelihood of emotional upsets. However, as a rule, you don't have control over other people and events. Trying to control the uncontrollable is a sure-fire recipe for drumming up more anxiety. Practicing watching your uncontrolled breath helps you to let go of your need to control things. Instead, you learn to simply allow things to be as they are. This is the essence of the Acceptance Tool work that you'll read about in chapter 19, Expectation Versus Reality.

Just as you noticed in the Body Scan Meditation, distractions will arise that pull you away from your breath. It doesn't matter what type of thoughts pop up; their content is not important for this practice. What is important is that you become aware that your attention has shifted away from the breath. Each time you notice a distraction and successfully come back to your breath, commend yourself on another mindful victory.

It can be frustrating noticing how often your mind wanders. Many beginners take their mind-wandering as evidence that they cannot meditate at all and give up. Please remember that it is perfectly normal for your mind to wander. Most people can't focus for even a minute without being distracted.

When you self-correct distractions, be gentle, yet firm. Be *gentle* in that you do not berate yourself for your wandering mind. Just kindly note the distraction. However, be *firm* by returning to the breath as soon as you notice that your mind has wandered. Sometimes the distracting thoughts will be more interesting than the breath, and you will be tempted to indulge in the distraction. This will hamper your attention training. As with any learning, consistency is critical.

When I was training my dog, Sophie, how to sit, I would say, "Sophie, sit," and she would sit for a moment or two before her puppy brain got distracted by some smell or sight. I would repeat, "Sophie, sit," and she would return and sit. Over time, with consistent training, she was able to stay for longer periods without succumbing to distractions. If I had been inconsistent in my training and sometimes just let her wander, then the training would have been less effective, and she may never have learned to be the well-behaved companion she is now.

Training your brain to manage distractions can make you more efficient and productive in your daily life. Research with Buddhist monks with tens of thousands of hours of meditation practice has demonstrated that attention training from meditation significantly improves attention skills and alters the brain networks that underlie attention.[14] But you needn't practice ten thousand hours to get benefits. Studies have shown that after just a few weeks of practice, changes in the brain can improve your attention and productivity.[15]

PRACTICE

You can follow the guided meditation on this books website (http://www.newharbinger.com/48817—audio accessory 4: Awareness of Breath) or use the instructions here. Find a comfortable seat and begin to feel the breath passing through your nose. As you focus on the breath sensations, your mind will be pulled by other thoughts, sounds, or body sensations. Just note them—*Thinking, Hearing,* or *Feeling*—and then return to focus on your breath.

One optional technique that may help you focus is counting your breaths. Count one for a breath in and out, then two for the next breath in and out. Only count up to ten, then repeat one to ten. This way, you won't get burdened by the numbers—*Inhaling 268, exhaling 268*—and can instead focus on the breath sensations. Remember that counting is optional.

Set a timer for five minutes. Remember to be gentle with yourself when your mind wanders but firm in bringing your attention back to your breath as soon as you notice the distraction.

SUMMARY OF THE BREATHING TOOL

So far, you've learned that short, rapid breathing turns up anxiety and that slow, deep breathing calms it down. You practiced using *ujjayi* belly breathing to establish a smooth, deep breath that reduces anxiety. You learn how to calm yourself further using Relaxation Breathing and the Bee's Breath. Finally, you began using Awareness of Breath to develop your attentional skills so that you can work better with time-wasting and anxiety-producing distractions.

Remember to be patient as you train yourself to breathe better. Probably the hardest thing about these Breathing Tools is remembering to use them. Since you do not yet have the habit of breathing deeply when you feel anxious, it requires more effort on your part to remember. To help, I recommend practicing each technique regularly. Daily practice will put the Breathing Tools at the top of your toolbox, so they're easier to access when you get anxious. Second, try providing reminders for yourself. For example, slap a sticky note on your desk at work or on your fridge or bathroom mirror that says, "Breathe." Finally, set intentions for yourself: "When I feel anxious, I will take five slow belly breaths," or "When I feel anxious, I will practice Relaxation Breathing for one minute." Setting clear intentions will create a mindful map of how you can manage your anxiety using these new breathing techniques.

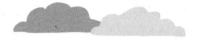

The Grounding Tool

When lost in anxious thoughts, you easily become dissociated from your body and your surroundings. Common idioms point to this dissociation, like "jumping out of your skin" and "being on the edge of your seat." One remedy for breaking the cycle of anxious thinking and calming your fight-or-flight arousal is to bring attention to your body and its connection to the immediate surroundings. This practice is called "grounding." By turning your attention away from the thoughts that fuel anxiety, you can step down from high-adrenaline states. Becoming more *physically* grounded helps you become more *emotionally* grounded. You feel more centered and therefore less perturbed by the storm of life swirling around you.

While working on the Observer Tool, you likely noticed how often anxious thoughts were oriented in the future. For example, worrying about delivering a presentation, looking stupid in front of your friends, or having enough money for retirement. The result is that you get overwhelmed in the present by something that may not happen for weeks, years, or …ever. Mark Twain reportedly said, "I've experienced a lot of tragedy in my life—most of it never happened."

Grounding pulls you out of future-oriented worries by drawing you back into the here and now. It reminds you to focus on managing what's on your plate today, not on all the plates stacked up in your future. Anyone would be overwhelmed trying to juggle all their future plates. On the other hand, when you come back to the present, you can usually manage what's happening now. Explicitly acknowledging to yourself that you are okay *now* calms your fear brain.

Grounding, much like breathing, is a practice that can be done anywhere and at any time. Whether you are in a meeting, driving down the freeway in traffic, or waiting in line at the store, it's easy to apply one of the following grounding techniques.

14. Touching the Earth

In the Touching the Earth practice, you simply notice where you are touching the earth. You can practice this technique anywhere, from an airplane to an elevator; you don't literally have to be touching the earth. Just notice where your body is resting on a surface. When standing, feel your feet. When sitting, feel your butt and your feet. When lying down, feel whatever body parts are touching the surface you're lying on—on a hard surface, it might be the back of your head, your upper back, your butt, and parts of your arms and legs; but on a soft surface, like a bed, much more of your body would be in contact with the surface.

Touching the Earth provides a fast and simple way to come back to the present. Take a moment now. Close your eyes and feel where you are touching down. Invite a long exhale, like a sigh, to help your body settle a little bit more into those surfaces. How does it feel to be grounded right here?

Grounding Feet. Grounding Feet is a technique similar to Touching the Earth, but it focuses on specific grounding points in your feet. You can practice this while standing or sitting. Shift your attention to feel sensations in these four corners on the bottom of your feet: the ball of the big toe, the ball of the pinky toe, the outer heel, and the inner heel.

Take a moment to feel the four corners one at a time in your left foot and then your right foot. In our shoe-wearing culture, we stuff our feet into shoes and ignore them. Despite this habitual disregard, you can reawaken your awareness to feel how your feet connect to the earth. Barefoot practice will make it easier for you to feel your feet connected to the floor or ground. Plus, research has found that barefoot walking on the earth can produce immediate improvements on a number of health-related factors, like reduced muscle tension and pain, lowered stress and anxiety, improved sleep, and enhanced immune function.[16]

15. Sensing Your Body

While the Touching the Earth practice is the most obvious type of grounding, you can also ground yourself by attending to other perceptual cues in your environment. I recommend three Sensing Your Body practices that ground you within yourself.

Five-Senses Grounding. This practice invites you to experience the present moment through each of your five senses. Let's try. One at a time, can you name something in your immediate surroundings that you see? Hear? Feel? Smell? Taste?

Sometimes, trying to find the right name for things sends you deeper into thinking and away from the direct sense of seeing, hearing, or smelling. For example, if you hear a bird singing, you might try to remember what type of bird it is, and then start thinking about when you last saw that bird or try to remember facts about its habitat or mating cycles. All of that thinking about the bird leads you further away from the present-moment experience of hearing the bird. If this happens, note to yourself, *Thinking,* and come back to simply hearing the bird. It's also fine to practice without naming everything you notice. For example, you could just hear the birdsong without mentally labeling it, *Birdsong.*

You can also just stay with one of these perceptual modalities. For example, let's try a listening meditation. Close your eyes and open your ears. Allow whatever sounds are in the environment to come into your awareness. Try not to push away some sounds or cling to others. Try not to judge the sounds. Simply be with whatever you hear.

Grounding Body Scan. When you're anxious, your body holds nervous tension that keeps you on the ready to deal with potential threats. This muscle tension is ungrounding. In this Grounding Body Scan Meditation, you scan through your body in the same way you did in the first Body Scan. However, instead of simply feeling your body as you scan through, you use your breath to help release tension from that body part to allow it to ground. For example, as you focus on your left arm, you inhale and feel the left arm. As you exhale, you allow the arm to release more deeply on the floor. You can guide yourself following the sequence described in chapter 7, or you can use a guided meditation on this book's website (http://www.newharbinger.com/48817—see audio accessory 5: the Grounding Body Scan Meditation).

Forward Folding. Another yogic approach to grounding involves Forward Folding poses. As you might guess, these involve folding your body forward at the hips. Forward Folding activates your brain's rest and digest system to counter anxious arousal. Keep in mind that you do not have to have any experience with yoga or be flexible to benefit from this technique. As a simple example, sit in your chair and let your torso lean forward toward your lap. Relax your neck and rest your forearms on your legs (or let your arms dangle on either side of your legs). Don't worry about how far you fold and don't strain to fold further. Just go to where your body takes you and rest there. Make sure you can breathe smoothly.

One caveat for these folds involves the safety of your lower back. It's better not to hang all of your torso weight onto your lower back. For example, in a standing forward fold, letting all of your head and torso weight hang down could potentially strain your lower back. To fold safely, take a deep breath into your belly to create a round inner tube of breath. Then brace by hugging the muscles of the front and side belly into the inner tube. It can also help to use your hands on your legs, blocks, or a wall to help bear the torso's weight. Avoid excessive rounding of your lower back, especially if you have any back problems or bone density issues.

This book's website (http://www.newharbinger.com/48817) has a worksheet, called Forward Fold Yoga Poses, that has photos demonstrating these poses: Half Splits, Wide-Legged Standing Forward Fold, Single-Leg Seated Forward Fold, Standing Forward Fold, Seated Forward Fold, Standing Forward Fold Using a Wall, Legs up a Wall, Recline Knee to Chest. Hold each pose for at least five slow breaths.

16. Soothing Touch

The yoga tradition describes a number of energy flows through the body. The upward flow, *prana vayu*, activates your nervous system, whereas the downward flow, *apana vayu*, sedates it. The two practices described here, Grounding Self-Massage and Submerging in Water, use this *apana vayu* to soothe your system.

Grounding Self-Massage. In this practice, you initiate the downward flow with slow massage strokes to help calm your nervous system. And who doesn't love a nice little massage? To try it out, you can use the guided meditation (http://www .newharbinger.com/48817—audio accessory 6: Grounding Self-Massage) or the instructions below. Of course, it's nicer when someone else is doing the massaging, but in days of quarantine, sisters are doing it for themselves.

Arms. To begin, sit comfortably, cross your arms, and place your hands on opposite shoulders. Slowly glide your hands down your arms from shoulders to elbows. Once at the elbows, hop the hands back to the shoulders, and repeat gliding down to the elbows. Repeat five strokes. Avoid stroking up from elbows to shoulders. Then, stroke from elbows to wrists a few times. Next, start again at the shoulders, and glide your hands down the whole length of the arm from shoulder to wrist. Repeat five strokes.

Chest. Stack your hands on your upper chest, and slowly glide them down the front of your chest to your low belly. Repeat five chest-to-belly strokes. Focus on how this feels, and let go of any thoughts that distract you from feeling.

Legs. Place your palms on your upper thighs close to the hip crease. Glide your hands down your legs to your knees. Replace the hands back on the upper thighs, and repeat five slow strokes. Next, stroke down from knees to shins, ankles, or feet, going only as far as you can comfortably reach as you lean forward. After five repetitions, move your hands back to your upper thighs, and stroke down the whole length of the leg five times. Once you've finished stroking the whole leg, sit upright with your palms facing down on your lap. Rest and notice the effects of the massage.

Submerging in Water. The natural element of water can activate your rest and digest system so that you feel calmer and more grounded.[17] You can simply run your hands under the faucet to feel the touch of the water on your skin, or you can take a shower and focus on the feeling of the warm water pouring over you. Submerging your body in water more completely, with a bath, hot tub, or swim, will further enhance the grounding effect. Sensory deprivation float tanks have been shown to reduce anxiety and create a deep sense of relaxation.[18] In these tanks, your body floats effortlessly in water that is heated to skin temperature and nearly saturated with salt to maintain your buoyancy. If you have access to a float center, I highly recommend the experience.

17. Walking Meditation

Walking is one of the most over learned habits in your behavioral repertoire, such that you can walk without needing to concentrate on it. But in the Walking Meditation, you turn your attention to walking, becoming aware of the sensations, movements, and balance of your body as it walks.

This grounding practice gives you another opportunity to work on your Observer Tool. When you become distracted, you'll practice refocusing on the present moment. You can use the guided meditation (http://www.newharbinger.com/48817 —audio accessory 7: Walking Meditation) or follow the instructions below.

Start by standing still and feeling the bottoms of your feet connecting with the ground. Once you are aware of your body standing, begin to transfer weight onto one foot, letting the other foot to step forward slowly. Feel it as it lands. Continue in this manner, taking slow, deliberate steps and feeling the feet touch down as you walk. After taking ten to fifteen steps, pause, standing still, and feel both feet on the ground. Then turn around and begin to walk again.

Start out by walking for only ten minutes. As you walk, you will inevitably get distracted. When that happens, note the distraction and pause for a moment. Then, from standing still, begin walking again.

Mantra Option. You can add a mantra to help you concentrate. For example, you can repeat, "swing, step," to reflect the swinging and stepping of each foot in sequence. Your verbal brain centers tend to distract you with an internal dialogue. Giving them something to do related to walking will decrease the likelihood of them distracting you with random thoughts.

18. Grounding in Nature

Grounding is especially effective when done in nature. Though we live in a digital age and spend a good chunk of our days staring at screens, humans have spent the largest slice of our evolutionary history living in close connection with nature. Our migration to crowded urban environments is still relatively new. While our animal bodies are adapting to these new conditions, they still feel most at home outdoors.

Our separation from nature is increasing. There are now more urban dwellers than rural dwellers, and today's children spend less time playing outside compared to previous generations.[19] People living in developed nations spend virtually all of their time indoors.[20]

Research in the scientific field of ecotherapy has demonstrated that spending time in nature reduces anxiety. People who are more connected to nature experience more positive emotions, vitality, and life satisfaction compared to those less well connected.[21] People who live near green spaces like parks or rural landscapes show better physical and mental health.[22]

In response to a public health epidemic of stress-related illnesses, the Japanese Forest Department developed the concept of *forest bathing*. The practice involves bringing your awareness to your senses while in a forested environment. This is akin to doing the Five-Senses Grounding Meditation while you're out in nature—walking and paying attention to what's around you. Studies have shown that forest bathing can stabilize your blood pressure, reduce stress hormones, and strengthen your immune system.[23]

The practice of earthing, making direct contact to the earth, is associated with enhanced immune function and reduced pain and stress.[24] Since your body is composed of mostly water and minerals, it is a great conductor of electricity. Direct contact with the electrons from the earth's surface balances your body's electrical charge. However, since our modern plastic- and rubber-soled shoes shield us from the earth's electromagnetic field, we live like cut flowers, disconnected from the earth's healing energy. To receive more benefit from earthing, it helps to walk barefoot or lie down in the grass or on a beach.

Being in nature also ignites a nearly automatic mindfulness, as we are predisposed to be captivated by natural beauty. Simply listening to the breeze in the trees, feeling the touch of sun on your skin, or smelling the scents of nearby flowers all easily draw you right into the here and now. So get outside. Mother Nature may be your best friend in managing your anxiety and helping you reconnect to a sense of well-being.

SUMMARY OF THE GROUNDING TOOL

Anxiety is ungrounding. When you are reexperiencing a past trauma or simply lost in anxious thoughts, you become dissociated from your body, your surroundings, and the events happening around you. Grounding practices help you return to the here and now by shifting your attention to your body's physical connection to the earth or to your sensory experience of your immediate environment. By returning to the present moment, you often find that things are okay now. Consciously becoming aware of feeling okay helps reduce your anxiety. Being in nature has an innate way of grounding and calming you. People who are more connected to nature are healthier, less anxious, and more content.

Step outside. Take a deep breath of fresh air. See what you see and feel what you feel. It only takes a moment to ground yourself in the here and now.

The Acceptance Tool

Joan is the mother of three elementary-school-aged boys. Her family had planned to go trick-or-treating together, but when it came time to leave, Joan's husband called to say that he was stuck at work and wouldn't be able to make it. So Joan and the boys set out without him. However, as they traipsed from house to house, Joan was stewing in anger, judging her husband for not being there. Her mind dredged up other examples of when he had failed to show up for their family.

As the boys gleefully continued collecting candy, Joan's mindful practice kicked in, and she noticed herself stuck wishing things were different than they were. This is a classic anxiety-producing scenario: feeling like life should unfold according to your plans and getting upset when it doesn't.

Recalling her tools, Joan tried to accept that her husband wasn't there. With that acceptance, her attention shifted to hear the boys' high-pitched giggles. She could see how much fun they were having with their costumes and candy. In her angry brooding, their antics had gone unnoticed. As she began to engage with the boys, her spirits lifted considerably. Later she told me how stunned she was by the dramatic difference acceptance had made.

But Joan's story is also a good reminder that acceptance of the moment doesn't mean resigning yourself to remain stuck in an anxiety-producing situation. In fact, Joan used her insights from observing her reactions to her husband's repeated absences to realize that the relationship wasn't working for her. She ended up getting a divorce the following year.

Acceptance makes the moment easier to navigate and provides clarity for how best to deal with problems, but it doesn't mean that you capitulate to the circumstances and stay stuck in something that isn't right for you.

As Joan's story reflects, when you fight what's happening, you not only rouse your anxiety, but you also miss out on the beauty of other things that are happening. When you resist or try to control life, you add suffering. When you accept life, you build more contentment. The feeling of not having control is a prime ingredient that feeds your anxiety. More people die from car accidents than they do from terrorism, but they are more anxious about terrorism because it is out of their control.

Mindfulness teaches you to be open and friendly with whatever comes your way. The poet Dorothy Hunt puts it this way.[25]

Do you think peace requires an end to war?
Or tigers eating only vegetables?
Does peace require an absence from
your boss, your spouse, yourself? …
Do you think peace will come some other place than here?
Some other time than Now?
In some other heart than yours?

Peace is this moment without judgment.
That is all. This moment in the Heart-space
where everything that is is welcome.
Peace is this moment without thinking
that it should be some other way,
that you should feel some other thing,
that your life should unfold according to your plans.

Peace is this moment without judgment,
this moment in the Heart-space where
everything that is is welcome.

I love the profound simplicity of "peace is this moment without judgment." The practice of acceptance is intertwined with one of the basic tenets of mindfulness. It is not so much other people and experiences that cause your anxiety, but rather your reactions to those people and experiences. While you can't control other people or your experiences, you do have some control over how you respond to them. The Greek philosopher Epictetus pointed this out more than two thousand years ago. He wrote that "we are disturbed not by things, but by the views which we take of them. Therefore, when we are disturbed or grieved let us never impute it to others, but to ourselves."[26]

19. Expectation Versus Reality

One of your brain's main jobs is creating expectations about what will happen based on your experience from the past. For example, when you read "twinkle, twinkle, little _____," your brain automatically fills in "star." It's quick, like a reflex, so that you hardly notice that your brain is filling in what it expects to hear. One recipe for anxiety is when reality doesn't match what your brain predicts. The greater the mismatch, the greater the anxiety.

One means of reducing anxiety is to accept reality as it is and to let go of your expectation of how you think it should be. One of my students exemplified this in dealing with her frustration with tulip growing. While planting the bulbs each fall, Cynthia enjoyed imagining what spring would bring. However, each spring, the tulip display never matched what she had envisioned. Some bulbs didn't grow due to the soil quality; others were gobbled up by industrious gophers. And every time Cynthia gazed out on her garden, she would feel disappointed and berate herself for not cultivating the tulips she had intended. The next fall, she would replant those that had not come up, only to be disappointed the following spring.

Using her mindful tools, Cynthia first realized how much upset her tulip garden was creating. Though it may not be a big deal for many, she invested a lot of her time and energy into her garden. Working with Acceptance, she began to notice times when her frustration over the poor tulip turnout appeared. With awareness, she was able to accept her frustration and then return to accepting the tulip garden as it was. When she wasn't focused on disappointment, she could pay more attention to the beauty of the existing tulips instead of obsessing about the missing ones. Acceptance helped reestablish her enjoyment of gardening. Then, last fall, Cynthia decided to foil the gophers by planting all of her bulbs in pots. Come spring, sure enough, she was rewarded with her biggest tulip display ever.

How are your expectations about how the world should run making you more anxious? How does it feel when you let go of the idea of "should" and embrace how things actually are? What actual things are you missing when obsessing about what you think *should* be happening?

20. Resistance to Acceptance

When you try to resist experiences, you add more conflict to an already difficult situation. Conversely, when you meet the world with acceptance, you add more ease, even amid difficulty.

Since the habit of struggling against your experience is so well ingrained, applying the Acceptance Tool is challenging. Acceptance may seem like you are resigning yourself to being stuck indefinitely in unpleasantness. This is how Chris felt.

With the blooming trees and fresh grass of spring comes an abundance of pollen, to which Chris is allergic. He reported feeling sorry for himself over his congested sinuses, sore throat, itchy eyes, headaches, achy muscles, and fatigue. He said he had been worried about his ability to teach his spin classes with his ratchety voice and faucet nose. "Snot dribbling onto my biking gloves is just not an inspiring look." He realized that he was catastrophizing how bad it would be but felt lost in self-pity.

Illness provides a challenging place to practice acceptance, because your knee-jerk responses are aversion and avoidance.

You may even wonder, *Why would I want to accept illness, when all I really want is for it to go away?*

It is important to remember that acceptance is not resignation. For example, with Chris's allergies, I reminded him that accepting his allergic reactions in the moment does not interfere with choosing to reduce his exposure to pollen, take allergy medicine, or clear his sinuses. Acceptance reduces your struggle with the experience while it's happening, so that you can move toward needed change from a place of peace, rather than from a place of frustration.

Acceptance also helps you feel more competent at handling things. On the other hand, catastrophizing can build up such an anxious storm that you feel overwhelmed by the experience, even by something as mundane as a runny nose. The feeling of *I can handle this* is critical in working with anxiety. When you think to yourself, *It's okay,* your mind has already begun to categorize your anxiety as something that is manageable, so it bothers you less.

PRACTICE

Continue to use the Observer Tool to notice your anxious symptoms, but now add accepting the symptoms. Remember that your anxiety is part of being human. Notice the habit of wanting to judge, control, or run away from your anxiety. Instead, notice the symptoms and let them be. For example, if you notice your jaw clenching, note, *Clenching jaw is here* (Awareness) and *It's okay that my jaw sometimes clenches* (Acceptance). With awareness and acceptance, you can choose to release the clenching jaw or not. We'll get to the Choice Tool next. For now, notice the impact of just shifting your attitude around clenching your jaw.

Take a moment to journal. What aspects of your anxiety are hardest to accept? Why do you think they are hard to accept? When you categorize your symptoms as physical, mental, emotional, or behavioral, which category is hardest for you to accept?

21. Willingness to Experience Anxiety

From seeing pictures of meditators looking so serene and unperturbed, you might get the idea that mindfulness meditation eradicates any difficult emotions from your life. Not true. You are still human. You will still get angry. You will still cry. You will still feel loss. You will still get silly. And you will still get anxious. Rather than eliminating emotions, mindfulness helps you relate to your emotions differently, so that they feel less overwhelming.

Our culture teaches us to suppress or ignore unpleasant emotions. Most movies and television shows depict unrealistic portrayals of life. Hollywood assures us too often that everything ends happily ever after. Even television commercials promote the idea that you should be happy 24/7. If not, then here's a pill you can take or a diet you can try.

From the time you first understand language, you are so bombarded by these unrealistically optimistic messages that the expectation of being happy seems like a birthright. So when unhappiness does arrive, as it does for us all, you think that something must be wrong. You may feel that you have to fix or hide your unhappiness in order to be normal. You may feel ashamed of your anxiety, and your shame causes you to suffer more.

Our cultural training also includes messages that it's not good to get overly emotional. Thus, you may try to suppress your negative moods or feel ashamed of them. And when suppressing negativity fails, you find ways to avoid difficult emotions: retail therapy, drinking, over exercising, or some other distraction.

The truth is that all emotions are a natural part of our human experience and are important for our survival. Anxiety is not a flaw in your human fabric, but a trait that helps you focus your attention to keep you alive. This is an inconvenient truth that most of us would rather ignore. However, resisting anxiety is a recipe for more suffering. Being willing to accept and experience your anxiety is what leads to relief.

The Indian guru Swami Satchidananda was an early importer of yoga to the West. He became well known after being the opening speaker at the Woodstock Peace Festival, and he later served as a spiritual adviser to many Hollywood stars. He used to say, "You can't fight the waves, but you can learn to surf."

Notice that same feeling with your anxiety. When you try to fight against your anxiety, the wave of anxiety can sweep you off your feet. In fact, research shows that the attempts to suppress painful emotions makes them occur more often, last longer, and cause more distress.[27] Also, trying to escape or forcibly suppress anxiety tends to increase your body's stress response. However, when you are willing to ride the ups and downs of your anxiety with compassion and kindness, you let go of the struggle and thereby create more ease.

I am a fan of the British sitcom *Absolutely Fabulous*. In the first episode of season three, Edina, in trying to placate her daughter, Saffy, tells her, "Lighten up, sweetie. Lighten up! You don't get things done just by being uptight, darling." I have clung to these words as a mantra, as they humorously encourage me to lighten up on my grip of how I expect other people to behave or how life events should unfold. When I "lighten up, sweetie," I have an easier time accepting what life throws my way.

22. Upgrading Acceptance to Appreciation

At first, just trying to accept life's challenges is hard enough. Your well-ingrained habits of avoiding unpleasantness makes the idea of accepting unpleasantness seem illogical. Nevertheless, it gets easier with practice, and you are rewarded with greater equanimity and peace.

One way of upgrading your Acceptance Tool is with appreciation. You not only allow life to be as it is, but you also choose to appreciate it. Appreciation is like acceptance on steroids.

Your brain has a hard time expressing both positive and negative emotions simultaneously. Studies have demonstrated that when appreciation goes up, anxiety goes down.[28] When you express gratitude, your brain releases dopamine and serotonin, two of the feel-good neurotransmitters that help shape your emotions. Further, people expressing appreciation have reductions in stress hormones and improved heart-rate variability,[29] a measure of rest and digest function that you'll learn about in chapter 40.

Acceptance and appreciation sound great, of course, but how do you suddenly develop the ability to be accepting and grateful? Practice! And you don't have to make it complicated. Take, for example, writing a thank you note. In one study, nearly three hundred college students who were seeking mental health counseling at their university were randomly assigned to three groups.[30] All of the groups received counseling, but the first group was also instructed to write one letter of gratitude a week for three weeks. The second group wrote about their thoughts and feelings around negative experiences. The third group did no extra writing.

Twelve weeks after the intervention, the folks who wrote the appreciation letters reported better mental health than the other two groups. This held true whether the grateful group sent their letters or not.

Further, the researchers invited some of the participants back three months later to participate in a brain-imaging study.[31] While in an fMRI scanner, participants completed a pay-it-forward task in which they were repeatedly endowed with an imaginary monetary gift and then asked to pass it on to a charitable cause to the extent they felt grateful for the gift.

The fMRI results revealed differences between the grateful-letter writers and those who didn't write letters. It is remarkable that simply writing three thank-you letters was associated with greater neural activation in gratitude and empathy circuits a full three months later. It appears that even simple gratitude practices can have long-lasting effects on your brain and psychological well-being.

PRACTICE

Cultivating appreciation is easy and feels great. Here are some simple techniques to get you started.

- Write thank-you notes.

- Write an appreciation letter to someone who has helped you at some point in your life.

- Daily Gratefuls: every night before you go to sleep, take a moment and reflect on the things that you appreciate from the day.

- Go out in nature and appreciate beauty.

- Be generous with thanking people who serve you during the day—the check-out person at your grocery store, a waiter, a bank teller, a Lyft driver, a teacher, an author.

- Try to see the benefit of difficult situations. Is there a lesson to learn? Is there guidance on how to improve the situation? Is there clarity on what to do next time?

- Appreciation Body Scan. Scan through your body, as you did earlier. As you focus on each body part, think of the ways it supports you. Be thankful for the help it provides. *Thank you, legs, for dancing me through this day. Thank you, tongue, for tasting that delicious meal.*

SUMMARY OF THE ACCEPTANCE TOOL

Now you have begun to learn how to become aware of your anxious symptoms and to accept them as they are. When you resist life, you add more struggle to what may already be a difficult situation. When you accept life, you develop more ease around what is happening. Accepting anxiety is challenging, because you typically see it as something wrong that needs fixing. Being willing to experience your anxious symptoms, rather than run away from them or repress them, makes them less uncomfortable. You develop the capacity to tolerate challenging emotions instead of feeling overwhelmed by them. You can upgrade your acceptance game by appreciating what life brings you, understanding that lessons can be gleaned even from your most trying experiences.

The Choice Tool

Now we come to the last tool in creating a mindful minute: choice. First, you become *aware* of what is happening in the moment. Second, you *accept* what you have noticed. Finally, you *choose* where to place your attention. What thoughts, words, or actions best align with your intentions for that moment?

Anxiety can be a time-consuming and unpleasant distraction. Think how often you spin your wheels, worrying about getting a job done instead of actually doing something that would help get it done. Consider how much time you waste fretting over future scenarios, many of which never end up happening anyway. Worrying and fretting not only waste your time, but they are also unpleasant mental places to spend your time. The Choice Tool is critical in redirecting your attention away from anxious thinking, allowing you to be more efficient in how you expend your energy.

One challenge that comes with the Choice Tool involves deciding where to put your attention now that you're aware. In working with anxiety, you might choose to apply one of your calming tools, like the Breathing or Grounding Tools. You can have a default plan: "When I feel anxious, I'll take three slow, deep breaths."

Another choice is to return to whatever you were doing before becoming distracted by your anxious thoughts. Maybe you were reading and return to the book, watching television and return to the show, or working and return to the task. The choice to return to what you were doing before provides an easy way to get started using the Choice Tool. You think, *What was I just doing? Ah, yes. Let me get back to that.*

However, that moment of choice provides a juncture more powerful than just returning to the status quo. It provides a window of opportunity for you to realign what you *are* doing with what you *want* to be doing in your life. Of course, you could go back to scrolling through social media when you stop worrying. But is endless scrolling really what you want for yourself in the long haul? You can use the power of choice to step away from unwanted habits. It does take effort to override the pull of comfortable habits, but that effort is worth it. It feels great to be doing things that align with your life's purpose. To get the most out of your Choice Tool, it helps to prepare by setting intentions ahead of time.

23. Intentions Help Direct Your Choices

Mary Wollstonecraft Shelley wrote, "Nothing contributes so much to tranquilize the mind as a steady purpose—a point on which the soul may fix its intellectual eye." Intention is the determination to act in a certain way—to have resolve. Working with intention requires resolve, especially when your intentions are at odds with long-held habits or at odds with what others around you are doing. One way to start working with intentions is to create more *general* intentions that apply to a broad range of circumstances. I'll share an example of one that has helped me.

During my first session of training to become a yoga teacher, we were studying the ethical principles of yoga. I was drawn to the second principle, truthfulness. I realized that from living as a closeted gay man for many years, I had developed a habit of being deceitful. In an environment that was extremely homophobic, I feared for my safety and was anxious about losing family and friends if anyone discovered I was gay. I lied about whom I spent time with, whom I was attracted to, and what I did in my free time. I was also trying to act more masculinely in order to fit in. We all have various social masks that we put on in order to make ourselves more acceptable, some more disingenuous than others. But over time, lying became a habit that slowly seeped into areas of my life unrelated to being gay.

While meditating on truthfulness, I recognized that lying didn't resonate with the trustworthy person I wanted to be. So I decided to stop lying. But despite my intention to speak only the truth, I kept lying. Habits are sticky things.

Nevertheless, with patient practice, I rebuilt the habit of truthfulness. First, I set an intention to replace falsehood with truth whenever I noticed I was lying. This was sometimes embarrassing, as when I had to admit to someone that I had just lied to them. And honestly, sometimes the fear of embarrassment won, and I didn't correct the lie. But generally, the feeling of realigning with the truth was worth the temporary embarrassment of fessing up to a lie. It was freeing not to be burdened with lies or by the anxiety that came from trying to remember which lie I had told to whom or the anxiety that came from not being okay being myself. By adopting one general intention, *Be honest*, I was able to upgrade many aspects of my life while at the same time cutting my anxiety in half.

Intentions can also be applied to more *specific* situations. For example, one of my students, Grace, was feeling anxious about her difficulty in getting pregnant. She wanted to eat more healthfully and stop drinking alcohol to improve her fertility. But since she was socially anxious, she drank on her Friday outings with friends in order to relax and enjoy her time with them. At the bar, she would rationalize that she wasn't pregnant yet and that since she wouldn't be able to drink once she was pregnant, having a drink now would be all right.

I guided her to set a more specific intention. Instead of thinking of avoiding alcohol, I asked her what she wanted to drink that aligned with her fertility goals. As a rule, it helps to frame your intentions in a positive light instead of avoiding behaviors you don't want. Grace decided that she would ask for seltzer with lime when the time came to order drinks. On a subsequent visit, she told me that she was surprised by how easy it had been to skip the adult drinks, having made a specific plan on how to navigate the moment when her impulse to drink was strongest.

Using intentions reaffirms your ability to create your experience. Though you are clearly influenced by your past, you do not have to be a victim of your past choices and habits. The present moment has magic in it, as it always gives you the opportunity to choose something new. That is why present-moment awareness is so central to your mindfulness training.

PRACTICE

Pick a general intention—like truthfulness, kindness, or appreciation—that you would like to apply to your life. Take time to select one that feels right to you, something that aligns with the person you aspire to be.

Then choose a specific event this week at which to practice your intention. Explore how the intention affects your experience. Remember that this is a practice and that habits are strong. Accept that your habits may initially override your intention. This is expected. But with patient practice, even well-ingrained habits can be uprooted.

24. Working with Habits

Since you are a creature of habit, your days are filled with a series of habits. Think of how routinized the first part of your day usually is: the way you brush your teeth and wash your face, get dressed, make breakfast, and commute to work.

As a rule, habits are enormously helpful, because they free up your brain to concentrate on things beyond shoe tying and egg scrambling. Imagine if you had to concentrate on every detail of washing dishes or driving your car. You'd burn so much mental fuel on the small stuff that you would be too exhausted to engage in more complex pursuits. William James wrote that "the more of the details of our daily life we can hand over to the effortless custody of automatism, the more our higher powers of mind will be set free for their own proper work."[32]

Though we usually think of habits as physical behaviors, you also have mental and emotional habits. For example, anxious minds tend to be judgmental minds, so you may have a habit of being judgmental. You do not have to consciously try to drum up a judgment; it is so routine that it pops into your mind, and sometimes out your mouth, without consideration. With emotions, you may have the habit of getting angry. You do not consciously decide this—*Let me sit down and be angry about this for a while*—but nonetheless, anger arrives unbidden and chugs along under its own habitual steam.

Many of your automatic behavioral, mental, and emotional patterns were developed in childhood. As such, the rationale for these habits is based on a child's understanding and thus may be faulty. However, now that they have become ingrained as habits, you don't think about their underlying flawed logic. In mindfully observing your habits, you may discover that some don't align with what you believe as an adult. As children, my siblings and I left the water running while brushing our teeth. To us, growing up on a farm with our own well, water seemed like an endless resource. Only in college did I become aware of water conservation and realize that my wasteful habit was based on a childhood assumption about an endless supply of fresh water.

When your brain is running on automatic pilot, your habits determine what happens. Doing what you've done before is easy. It takes awakening to the present moment to make choices that differ from your habits. Viktor Frankl wrote, "Between stimulus and response there is a space. In that space lies our freedom and power to choose our response. In our response lies our growth and freedom."

Frankl was an Austrian physician, who in 1942 was deported with his family to a Jewish ghetto in Czechoslovakia. Later, he was moved to Auschwitz and suffered the dehumanizing conditions of the concentration camp. Though his wife and family were killed in the camp, Frankl survived. After the war he described his experience in his book, *Man's Search for Meaning.*[33] "Everything can be taken from a man but one thing: the last of the human freedoms—to choose one's attitude in any given set of circumstances, to choose one's own way."

Frankl attributes his survival to his ability to decide how to respond to the horrors of the camp. This harkens to one of the underlying precepts of mindfulness: it is not so much the circumstances or people that cause your stress and anxiety; it is your *reaction* to those circumstances and people that determines how you feel and what you do. Even when your outer circumstances seem hopeless, you have the power to choose how you respond to those circumstances in a way that can either increase or lessen their burden.

We are creatures of habits with our emotional lives, too. Can you think of a person in your life who always seems to push your buttons? You have probably developed the habit of reacting either with anxious withdrawal or defensive anger when this happens. You may want to break the cycle, but each time this person pushes your buttons, you find yourself reacting exactly as you have in the past. With mindfulness, you become aware of the moment after the person pushes your buttons (stimulus) but before you start anxiously reacting (response). In that space lies your power to choose a different response.

My student Julie found that space when working with a long-established habit that emerged when she felt judged:

> While I love my mom and get along with her most of the time, she tends to be hypercritical. Using the spaciousness that I have grown through my meditation, I can identify the moment when her critical comments hurt my feelings. I used to quickly snap back with a hurtful comment of my own or with angry silence. Using the Observer Tool, I am now more skilled at noting my reaction to her comments—*Wow, that hurt my feelings*—before I actually respond. I can pause in that space between her comment and my response, so I don't snap back with more negativity. In doing so, I've realized that her comments are really more about her experience and not intended to hurt me.

Admittedly, they still can sting, but I've learned to approach her with more compassion and less reactivity.

It may help to review your anxious habits by recalling the list of anxious symptoms you produced in the Observer Tool section. For example, an emotional habit common to people who suffer from anxiety is irritability.

Working with such habits requires patience. On one occasion, you may catch yourself before responding irritably and think how wonderful mindfulness is. On the next occasion, you might regress back into the irritable habit and conclude that this mindfulness crap is a waste of time. Changing habits is definitely not a one-shot proposition. Consider all of the years that you have been practicing the habit, driving it deeper and deeper into your habit brain. Accordingly, it takes time to unplug from one habit and to develop a new one. How much time? That is the million-dollar question, and there is no simple answer.

The "stickiness" of a habit depends on how long you have been practicing it, whether an emotional component is associated with it, and the context in which it emerges, as well as your personal motivation to change. Many self-help books claim you can change a habit in a mere twenty-one days.

That magical number evolved from a book written in 1960 by a plastic surgeon named Maxwell Maltz. He observed that after undergoing a surgical procedure, it took his patients a *minimum* of twenty-one days to adapt to their new circumstances, be it becoming used to phantom-limb pain after an amputation or adjusting to seeing their newly styled nose. His book, *Psycho-Cybernetics,* influenced a whole industry of self-help gurus to follow.[34] The oversimplification came when subsequent authors changed his suggested "*minimum* of twenty-one days" to just "twenty-one days." But realistically, twenty-one days is a minimum.

A better estimate comes from a recent study, which followed ninety-six participants over the course of twelve weeks as they attempted to develop a new everyday habit of their choice, like jogging.[35] Participants needed an average of sixty-six days before the new behavior became habitual. Variability between participants was high, as some learned their chosen behavior in as few as eighteen days, while others took an estimated 254 days. So moderate your expectations and be patient. It's not going to happen overnight.

25. Habits Are Driven by Context

You may be wondering, since habits are so automatic, what causes them to emerge when they do. Habits initially develop by gradually pairing behaviors with the contexts in which they occur.[36] For example, you may have the habit of having a cup of coffee in the morning with breakfast. The coffee drinking is paired with the temporal context (morning) and the situational context (breakfast). Contextual cues may include locations, times of day, people, preceding actions in a sequence, or other things.[37]

Your brain's executive centers coordinate learning the new behavior, but once the habit is established, its function is taken over by a more rudimentary part of the brain, the basal ganglia. The basal ganglia automatically produce the habit when the appropriate contextual cues are encountered. For example, the context of morning and breakfast automatically cues coffee drinking. Estimates suggest that over half of our daily activities are driven by this context-to-habit association.[38] But by knowing that context drives your habits, you can use context to help alter your habits.

You should recognize that habits that carry an emotional valence, like anxiety, are more firmly imprinted in your brain than behavioral habits, like jogging, and thus will take longer to shift. Be patient. It can be frustrating when you witness the reemergence of an old habit. You may feel as if your tools are not working, and you may want to abandon your efforts altogether. Animal research has reported that habits remain imprinted in the basal ganglia even after the behavior is extinguished, and thus they can reemerge if the right context is encountered.[39] This helps explain why it is so hard to permanently extinguish a habit.

PRACTICE

One habit that you may be trying to establish is a daily meditation practice. To help kick-start your practice, think of all the contextual cues associated with it. When does it happen? Where does it happen? What are you doing just before you start meditating? With whom does it happen? Once you have reflected on all of the contextual cues, try to be consistent. For example, practice at same time of day and in the same location. This will make it easier for your brain to establish the habit of meditation.

26. Behavioral Avoidance

One of the most common habits associated with anxiety is behavioral avoidance. If you imagine that an event may make you anxious, you avoid it. The behavior of avoiding certain places, people, or activities can become so habitual that it happens without your even noticing that you're doing it.

While it is natural to want to avoid the discomfort associated with anxiety, it is important to understand that the habit of behavioral avoidance can become problematic. When you avoid something, avoidance is reinforced, since it provides relief from the anxious symptoms you would have encountered. For example, if you are anxious about going to a party, you might choose not to go. By staying home, you don't experience social anxiety, and thus the habit of avoidance is reinforced.

In psychology, this is called "negative reinforcement": strengthening a behavior (avoidance) through the removal of an unpleasant stimulus (anxiety). When you notice the effectiveness of avoidance in one situation, you apply it in other anxiety-provoking situations. Over time, you get more and more sensitive to having any anxious reactions, and avoidance becomes your main strategy for coping with anxiety. Your world gets smaller and smaller as the number of acceptable activities, people, and situations diminishes. It's like "The Princess and the Pea." Instead of becoming more able to handle anxiety, you become hypersensitive to it. Even a hint of an anxious symptom makes you duck and cover.

In the extreme, anxiety sufferers go to great lengths to avoid anxiety. They end up feeling comfortable only in a limited number of safe and familiar contexts. With agoraphobia, people don't feel safe in public places and get stuck staying at home. Their anxiety is caused by fear that they may not be able to escape or manage their panic if a situation intensifies their anxiety. Overall, avoidance unleashed turns everyday worries into psychiatric disorders.

If you always kowtow to anxiety, your anxiety gets scarier and more powerful. On the other hand, if you courageously address your anxiety, you become more resilient to stressors and take back the power anxiety has over you. That is why it is important not to feed your habit of behavioral avoidance. Sure, you can get temporary relief by avoiding an anxiety-provoking situation, but it isn't worth the long-term harm of giving your anxiety more power. The idea of being stress-proof is not that you avoid stressors but, instead, that you learn to remain grounded and calm amid stressors.

To work mindfully with behavioral avoidance, you first need to become aware of it. Remember that habits occur automatically. Once you *notice* you are avoiding something, you *accept* that the habit has shown up in that moment. Then you *choose* whether it might be helpful to face the situation you are avoiding in order to build your resilience.

Keep in mind that in some cases, avoidance can be an appropriate strategy. Don't feel that you have to throw yourself into every situation that makes you anxious. We all have our limits, and it's important to honor your limits. Just be willing to test your limits—or else they'll keep growing more restrictive over time.

One way that behavioral avoidance shows up is through distraction. You may distract yourself with social media, television, books, food, drugs, gossip, shopping, cleaning, sex…any number of things. Mindful awareness helps you notice when you are engaged in distracting behaviors. With awareness, you can choose to continue distracting yourself, or you can choose to reengage in whatever activated the avoidance in the first place.

Avoidance can diminish your quality of life by limiting your access to people, places, and activities that may bring you joy. Avoidance can also be a measured response. For example, you may choose to go to a social gathering but not be fully engaged once there.

In my anxiety workshops, students are invited to engage purposefully in an activity that provokes anxiety so that they can practice using mindfulness to manage their anxiety. One student, Sarah, had been invited by a friend to a spa day in San Francisco. She normally would have made up an excuse to bow out of the spa trip. Instead, she decided to use the invitation as an opportunity to test out her mindful tools.

While Sarah was checking in at the spa, the greeter reviewed some of the guidelines. She informed Sarah that it was a clothing-optional facility that allowed alcohol on the premises. As these words sunk in, Sarah began to realize this wasn't the kind of spa she had envisioned. *Drunk naked people?* she thought, *I can't do this.*

She felt her heart start to pump more vigorously and noticed an impulse to bolt out the door to safety. Determined, though, not be run by fear, she started breathing deeply and continued to listen to the orientation. Soon enough, she was passing through to the changing rooms. Sarah noticed her discomfort with seeing all these naked strangers, but also noticed how they seemed comfortable being in the buff. *If they don't care, why should I?* she mused.

Sarah found her friend, Kelly, and, still feeling anxious, asked Kelly if she could change her massage appointment so they could leave earlier. Kelly checked, but the spa was fully booked. It would still be another two hours before Kelly's massage, so Kelly shrugged and said that they'd have to just chill and enjoy the place until then.

Chill? Enjoy?! *Survive, more like it,* Sarah thought, but then she returned to her mindful toolkit. *Just breathe. Just notice. It's okay. You've got this.*

As the minutes ticked on, Sarah began to acclimate to these new surroundings. She noticed that she was feeling less nervous and even enjoying her time with her friend. Having company made the situation bearable. But when Kelly's massage time arrived, Sarah realized she was going to have to fly in this steamy jungle of nakedness alone. Another surge of anxiety surfaced. She named her discomfort, took some deep breaths, and decided to explore. She found a hot tub, lightly populated with a couple of other spa-goers. Sarah girded her resolve, took a deep breath, and then plopped her naked self in with them. By the time Kelly's massage was done, Sarah was much more at ease with the whole scene. Her impulse to flee had passed, and she and Kelly ended up staying even longer.

The smile on Sarah's face in recounting her adventure was the best payment I could ask for as a teacher. Her story, and others like it, reflect our ability to engage in life, even when it's a little scary. When we listen to fear, we miss out on some of the delights life has to offer. When we accept our anxious symptoms, they become less noxious, and we are able to take advantage of opportunities that we would have otherwise missed.

Now, I think that Sarah's venture to the clothing-optional spa was akin to jumping into the deep end of the anxiety pool. I don't suggest that you start with something as extreme. A measured approach is more effective, and one you'll get to practice in the inoculation exercise in chapter 29.

Congratulations to Sarah and all of the other courageous students learning to face their fears. As Marianne Williamson wrote, "as we let our own light shine, we unconsciously give other people permission to do the same. As we are liberated from our own fear, our presence automatically liberates others."[40]

In your journal, write some example of choices you have made that were driven by the desire to avoid anxiety. Can you think of examples from work? In your relationships? With leisure activities? What are some of the costs of behavioral avoidance?

27. Choose to Be Here Now

We have all heard the catchphrase "Be here now," made famous by the same-titled book by Ram Dass.[41] Some people may discount the phrase as being too much associated with New Age spirituality, especially given that the author was an LSD-tripping, counterculture hippie. However, most spiritual traditions emphasize the importance of present-moment awareness in finding lasting contentment and well-being.

The idea of cultivating presence is what inspired Thoreau to hide away at Walden Pond. It underlies the "just for today" philosophies of addiction-recovery groups like Alcoholics Anonymous. The present moment is a place of power. You cannot change what happened yesterday. You cannot change what will happen tomorrow. However, you can direct your thoughts, words, and actions right now in a way that resonates with your intentions and values.

For those seeking a more science-driven justification for being present, a large-scale study by two Harvard psychologists found that being present leads to greater happiness.[42] In the Track Your Happiness study, 2,250 participants downloaded an app to their smartphones. The app notified them at random times throughout the day, posing three questions: What are you doing? What are you thinking? How happy are you? For the happiness prompt, they ranked themselves on a 100-point scale from miserable to ecstatic.

The authors assessed happiness under two basic conditions: on-task and mind-wandering. Participants were considered on-task when they were thinking about what they were doing. Participants were mind-wandering when they were thinking about something other than what they were doing.

Results showed that people rated themselves significantly happier when they were on-task. This was true even if they were doing boring activities or thinking of something that was more exciting than what they were doing. Again, mind-wandering was associated with being less content.

So you can build more happiness by practicing being present. It will help you to release your anxious ruminations about the future, and, who knows, you might notice something delightful happening right now.

SUMMARY OF THE CHOICE TOOL

Where you put your attention determines your experience of that moment. When your attention gets caught in anxious thoughts, you spend a lot of your time feeling miserable. Choosing to shift your attention away from anxious thoughts helps you feel more at ease and happy.

Establishing intentions for yourself provides a roadmap for navigating in-the-moment choices. Intentions can be general, like *Be kind,* to cover a broad range of circumstances, or they can be specific, like *Be kind to Mom when she makes disparaging comments,* to help you navigate particular situations.

Behavioral avoidance is one of the most common habits associated with anxiety. You naturally avoid things if you think they might make you anxious. However, the habit of avoidance can grow to unhealthy proportions, causing you to miss out on opportunities in your life. It takes courage to face something stressful rather than avoid it. And doing so empowers you to deal with stressors and builds your resilience against them. By contrast, always running away from stressors gives them more power, and you become more afraid of their potential harm.

People report being more content when they are present with what they are doing compared to when they are lost in thought. The present moment is the only time you have to choose where to place your attention to build the life that aligns with your values. Choose to be here now.

The Choose Your Story Tool

When you think about anxiety, it's usually with an attitude of *Ugh, Oh crap,* or *Why me?* You feel it is an impediment to being happy. You've noticed how anxiety spurs other reactions, like frustration and avoidance, which can make a difficult experience even worse. We've established that you can't control what life brings you. However, what you can control is whether you let yourself get lost in a negative story every time anxiety appears. Remember that anxiety itself is not the problem. Instead, your response to anxiety determines whether you make it a problem. Miles Davis once said, "It's not the note you play that's the wrong note—it's the note you play afterward that makes it right or wrong." In this section, you will take a look at how your story about anxiety impacts your experience of anxiety. If your story is making anxious moments worse, you can learn how to reinterpret anxiety to lessen its negative influence.

28. Reinterpret Your Body's Anxious Reaction

I grew up with a fear of the ocean, due in part to seeing the movie *Jaws* as an impressionable eight-year-old. Several years ago, I had the chance to swim in the open ocean with spinner dolphins. After a twenty-minute boat ride from shore, the time came to dive into this endless expanse of blue, and I panicked and froze. However, as I accessed my rational mind, I remembered that shark attacks are quite rare, especially around a pod of dolphins. I was able to reinterpret the physiological arousal I was experiencing as excitement. This new story allowed me to lean into the experience rather than shy away from it. I ended up absolutely loving my time with the dolphins. It was only afterward that I fully realized what I would have missed had I not been willing to question my anxious inner dialogue and dive in.

Like most people, you probably think that anxiety involves:

- panic, confusion, and upset

- fear of looking bad

- avoidance

- a heightened sense of vulnerability

However, a different interpretation of those same symptoms might involve:

- enhanced attention and perception

- improved clarity of purpose

- activated courage to face a challenge

In other words, your anxiety can be empowering rather than debilitating. When you anxiously avoid things, you miss out on valuable life experiences. But you don't have to let fear drive your life. Instead, lean into what excites you and courageously engage with life.

Let's look at another anxious story that could use some reinterpreting. When you're feeling anxious, it can seem like you're the only one bothered by anxiety. You've experienced how it interferes with your ability to do well, but at the same time, you think that other people are able to perform well because they don't get anxious. Fake news. Even pros with years of practice under their belts still get nervous. But professional athletes and musicians have learned to interpret their anxiety as a tool to muster their energy and hone their focus, whereas amateurs believe that their anxiety will leave them panicked and flustered.

One study beautifully demonstrated how reinterpreting your anxious symptoms can enhance your performance.[43] As a group of college students were about to take a practice version of the Graduate Record Exam (GRE), half of them were given a card that read: "People who feel anxious during a test might actually do better. Therefore, if you feel anxious during the practice test, you shouldn't feel concerned.… Simply remind yourself that your arousal could be helping you do well."

That was the entire intervention—just reading the advice to reinterpret their anxious symptoms. Despite its simplicity, the advice reaped big rewards. The students who read the card scored fifty points higher (out of eight hundred possible points) on the practice exam compared to those who did not. People spend a lot of money and time on prep courses to improve their GRE scores even a few points. So this fifty-point bump was certainly nothing to sniff at. Think where you might apply the advice that anxiety could help rather than hinder you: tests, interviews, dates? How does this idea change your relationship to that anxiety-provoking situation.

In the study, the researchers wondered if the students who read the card did better because the advice calmed them down. To test for this, they collected saliva samples to measure the stress hormones produced when you're anxious. It turned out that both groups had upticks in stress hormones related to their test-taking jitters. So it wasn't that those who read the card didn't get nervous. Instead, they were able to not let their anxiety get the best of them.

My student Anita reported how reinterpreting her anxious symptoms helped her with public speaking. She had a writing fellowship, and as part of the writing program, she was invited to give a public reading of her work. Since it would be her first time sharing her work in front of an audience, she got so nervous that she almost cancelled. But she recognized from her mindfulness training that her avoidance would only reinforce the habit of choosing from fear. She knew in her heart of hearts that she wanted to participate, even though the idea terrified her.

The night of the reading, Anita felt a lot of anxiety in her body. She worried that her anxiety would affect her ability to stand still and read. As she waited her turn, she practiced deep belly breathing and noted her symptoms, *Racing heart is here, Trembling hands are here, Shallow breath is here.* She tried to bring an attitude of acceptance to her symptoms but couldn't quite muster it. What did help was remembering that anxiety sensations mirror excitement. She told herself that she was feeling excited. This reinterpretation helped her to calm down enough to get through the reading. She ended up doing great and garnered many compliments from strangers hearing her work for the first time.

PRACTICE

Journal about the costs of trying to design an anxiety-free life.

- Can you identify choices you have made that likely were driven by the desire to avoid anxiety at work, in your relationships, or in leisure activities?

- Are there opportunities you have not pursued in those domains because of anxiety?

- What comes to mind about the ways in which you avoid people, places, or activities because of anxiety?

29. Inoculation

Ralph Waldo Emerson wrote, "Do the thing you fear, and death of fear is certain." This truism of how to become anxiety-proof relates to a technique called "inoculation." A medical inoculation exposes your body to a weakened virus or bacteria that is strong enough to trigger a response, but not so strong as to overwhelm your body. Inoculation to anxiety works the same way. You expose yourself to a situation that produces a manageable level of anxiety while applying your tools to ground and calm yourself. With practice, you build trust in your ability to manage anxiety whenever it shows up. Over time, with repeated success, your fear brain quiets, and your anxious symptoms diminish.

It's important to start inoculation with something that is manageable. If you start with the most terrifying thing on your list, you might inflict more trauma and further entrench your anxiety around that situation. My student Ainsley described how she broke down her fear of freeway driving into more manageable components for the inoculation practice:

> When I was little, my family was in a terrible car accident on a freeway entrance ramp. The accident made my whole family afraid to drive. In fact, my mom told

me never to drive. Despite her objections, I got my driver's license. But even after years of driving, freeway entries are still a big problem for me.

For the inoculation exercise, I was initially perplexed about how to find a manageable way to practice driving onto freeways, because anytime I would even approach a freeway, I panicked. So I decided to watch YouTube tutorials on how to safely enter a freeway. At first, just watching the YouTube clips made my breath stop and my muscles clench. But I stayed with it and practiced consciously slowing my breath and reassuring myself. When I did this, my anxiety lightened, and the tutorials became easier to watch.

After some success with the tutorials, I decided to try to drive onto a freeway. As I approached the entrance ramp, I noticed that I was holding my breath. I reminded myself to breathe deeply, like I had done during the YouTube videos. It worked! The drive ended up being fine. I was proud that I could take baby steps toward feeling more comfortable on the freeway ramps and pleased to find how effective the breathing tool was in reducing my driving anxiety.

PRACTICE

- Pick an activity that you associate with a mild amount of anxiety (in the ten to twenty range on a hundred-point scale). If you pick an activity that produces more anxiety, break it into smaller, more easily digestible components that evoke less anxiety, like Ainsley did with her freeway driving.

- Set aside time to engage in that activity.

- Use your Observer Tool to notice how you are feeling as you approach and engage in the experience. Accept whatever reactions you have, even if they include more avoidance or other anxious symptoms. Use Relaxation Breathing and Grounding to help you calm your system when you feel anxious.

- Repeat your practice experiment several times in order to train your fear brain to be less reactive to this situation.

30. Choose to Build Resilience

The inoculation practice is based on the aphorism, "That which doesn't kill you makes you stronger." By choosing to face your anxiety with courage, you become more emboldened to face life head on, even when anxious symptoms arise. If you always duck and cover when you feel anxious, you'll never develop the wherewithal to face life's challenges. Instead, you'll become more vulnerable to your anxious symptoms, and your life will be increasingly directed by fear.

The relationship between hardship and psychological resilience is not straightforward. As you might guess, adversity can lead to mental and emotional strife. Things like physical or sexual abuse, the death of a loved one, and homelessness are all associated with negative psychological outcomes.[44] However, what's interesting is that having no experience with adversity also leads to poor psychological outcomes.

In one study of 2,398 adults, those who reported a high number of negative life experiences showed increased stress and decreased life satisfaction.[45] However, those who reported *no* such experiences also showed increased stress and decreased satisfaction. So trying to design an adversity-free life is not the solution to being anxiety-free. In the study, it was the group who reported *moderate* hardship in their lives who experienced lower stress, lower functional impairment, and higher life satisfaction. In addition, those who had dealt with some prior adversity were better able to manage recent adversities.

Exposure to stress has a positive, toughening effect when the exposure is limited and includes a chance for the person to recover.[46] Resilience leaves you more able to manage difficult situations and helps you feel less anxious about your ability to handle future challenges.

Overall, the inoculation practice teaches you how to cope with stressful situations, to reinterpret the negative stories your fear brain repeats, and to build resilience against future stressors. Because it's hard to face things that make you nervous, you will likely want to avoid the inoculation practice. Notice avoidance, but remember: avoidance reinforces your fear of anxiety, while practicing inoculation builds your courage to face challenges. You choose.

PRACTICE

In a journal, write down at least three long-term benefits you hope to gain by doing your exposures. Perhaps you long to be able to take on new career-advancing projects. Maybe you want the voice in your head to whisper more empowering stories. Or perhaps you'd like to have the inner resources to respond better to life's emergencies. Reflect on the area of your life that might benefit from having resilience, and use this to motivate your practice.

31. To Struggle or Not to Struggle

When you're nervous, you often try to avoid or control what's happening—in other words, you struggle. Struggling with the situation happens automatically and can persist even after the troubling event that caused it has passed. What if you could learn to turn off your struggle?

Imagine that you have a "struggle switch" in your brain. When it is flipped on, you fight with whatever is happening.[47] This struggle might include trying to control other people, the situation, or your own reactions. When you're struggling, your anxious symptoms are harder to bear, and you compound your anxiety with secondary emotions. For example, you might feel angry at someone for making you anxious. You might feel ashamed for being anxious or berate yourself for letting anxiety get the best of you. The struggle switch acts like an amplifier for negative emotions, making a stressful situation more challenging.

Now imagine you could reach up in your brain and turn off the struggle switch. Here's how: instead of trying to escape or control the situation, simply allow it to be as it is. The moment may still be unpleasant, but you don't add to the unpleasantness. Instead, you let go of the struggle against it.

"Letting go" can have different connotations. You might imagine it like releasing a helium balloon, watching the problem gently drift away. However, letting go sometimes involves releasing something that doesn't immediately go away. Imagine your anxious thought as a marble you're holding in your fist, with your palm facing up. When you open your fingers to let go of the marble, it remains resting in your palm. Similarly, when you let go of your struggle, you loosen your grip on the situation and reduce your fight against it, but the problem, the troublesome life event, remains. So don't be disappointed if turning off your struggle switch doesn't immediately fix everything. Do notice how letting go softens your approach so that you can handle the situation with more ease.

PRACTICE

Think of something that has been worrying you lately. As an experiment, turn *on* your struggle switch and purposefully ramp up the ways you struggle against this experience. Are you trying to control or avoid someone, a situation, or your reactions? Notice how the struggle feels in your mind and body. Notice the stories of struggle in your internal dialogue. Journal about how you struggle with this situation.

Next, imagine reaching up and turning off your struggle switch. The issue may still be problematic, but you are choosing not to try to control it, fight against it, or run away from it. Allow the reactions you have to be just as they are. Then write about how it feels when you are not struggling.

Create a clear mental image of your struggle switch to help you become more adept at flipping it off at will. This week, use your Observer Tool to notice when your struggle switch is on. Become aware of it and accept it. Then practice turning it off.

32. Deprioritizing the Ego

Much of your anxiety comes from defending your ego. The ego is the psychological construct of yourself made up of all the experiences and preferences that make you uniquely you. The ego always wants to protect itself—it hates feeling ignored, judged, insulted, demeaned, or wronged.

Anytime your ego feels slighted, it will work to justify itself. You're prone to believe these justifications, in part because they pop up in your mind so quickly, but mostly because they reinforce the idea that you are right. The repair strategies that the ego uses include anger, defensiveness, self-justification, self-delusion, and blaming. When you notice these strategies, it's a sign that your ego is in self-defense mode.

For the ego, self-preservation is paramount. Even when you know that you've messed up, the ego is quick to rationalize the wrongdoing in order to maintain your sense of righteousness. It is easier to imagine that you are right than to accept the possibility that you have done something wrong. When you are blamed for something, notice how quickly your mind says, *but, but, but*…to rationalize whatever has happened and to free yourself of blame.

To work with the ego, begin with awareness. Observe when your ego jumps into self-defense mode. Accept that it is a natural reaction that all humans share. Choose to release any self-defensive behaviors and allow your ego to be diminished. This is truly next-level work, as it can feel like an attack to your sense of self. Be patient as you observe your reactions to deprioritizing the ego. By working with the Observer Tool and looking at the situation as a neutral witness instead of from the point of view of the ego, you realize that your awareness, which reflects your deepest essence, remains unscathed by the criticism to which the ego is reacting.

You can practice deprioritizing the ego further by watching for habits that boost your ego. For example, experiment with not trying to be the cleverest guest at a dinner party, the most balanced student in a yoga class, or the spouse who is always right. I know it can be hard. Just experiment! By bringing awareness to your ego, you will start to see how it fuels your anxiety and how, when you stop defending your ego, your anxiety declines.

A side benefit of deprioritizing the ego is that it makes it easier for you to connect with others. When you drop the "I'm right; you're wrong" story, you open to a shared humanity, seeing the rightness in others as well as your own imperfections. It allows you to find harmony with others, even when you have different social, political, or religious views. Through practice, you start to feel less anxious around people who are different than you. And in a world that seems more divisive than ever, your practice of deprioritizing the ego creates a ripple of connection that can help heal those divides.

PRACTICE

To work mindfully with the anxiety produced from a sensitive ego, apply the Observer Tool. When your ego is in self-defense mode, your habit may be to chastise yourself: *I shouldn't be so defensive* or *I can never seem to admit to doing anything wrong.* It doesn't help to judge your ego-based behaviors. Instead, when someone criticizes you, judges you, or blames you, try to pause. Watch as the ego jumps into self-defense mode. You can observe the defensive reactions—self-justification, blaming, and anger—without voicing them. Accept that the ego does what it does, just like the fear brain does what it does. You choose whether or not ego and fear drive your words and actions.

In moments of ego-defensiveness, you may feel uncomfortable or frustrated. Continue to observe yourself, allowing these transient emotions to be okay: *It's okay that I'm angry.*

You can also use your Observer Tool to notice times when you are trying to build yourself up in the eyes of others. Set an intention to refrain from self-aggrandizing activities. When you notice ego-driven thoughts or behaviors, try to deprioritize the ego.

PRACTICE

Journal about which stories, emotions, and body sensations arise when your ego feels attacked. How does it feel when you are bolstering your ego? What's it like when you purposefully choose to deprioritize the ego? Over time, you'll feel lighter and more joyful with less ego baggage.

SUMMARY OF THE
CHOOSE YOUR STORY TOOL

Whether or not your anxiety bothers you and interferes with your performance depends, in part, on the story you tell about anxiety. If you see it as an impediment to a happy and productive life, it's more likely to get in your way. However, when you follow the lead of professionals who have learned to use anxiety to their benefit, you too may find that it helps you feel energized and focused.

You can reframe your negative story of anxiety by inoculating yourself to situations that make you anxious. With practice, you learn that the catastrophic story your fearful brain tells is just that, a story. You find out that the things you fear are actually things you can manage. When you believe in your ability to manage stress, you reduce the power anxiety has over you and become more resilient to stress.

Another way we make anxiety bigger and scarier than it needs to be is by struggling against what life brings us. Trying to control a situation, other people, or your own reactions usually amps up anxiety. Letting go of struggle can help you accept the situation as it is—and accept yourself as you are.

This is difficult for the ego, which loves to stir up drama around difficult situations. But when you deprioritize the ego, you can reduce its anxiety-inducing drama and consequently feel more at ease. Finally, once your fear and ego stories start to quiet, you notice other inner voices—voices related to your intentions and values that help direct your choices. For example, you can choose to be guided by kindness.

The Kindness Tool

Emotions in our culture often get a bad rap. If someone says that you're "overly emotional," they're saying you're unstable or not thinking straight. We prioritize reason over emotion so much that it can seem like merely *having* emotions is wrong. You hear people claim that being angry is bad for your health. You see commercials advertising pills that will fix you if you're sad. And on and on. In a society that pathologizes emotions, it's easy to feel ashamed of your anxiety. Unfortunately, your shame only makes your anxiety worse.

One remedy for anxiety-related shame and self-criticism is kindness. By simply choosing to be kind to yourself in anxious moments, you can flip a switch, much like your struggle switch, that shifts you into a friendlier way of managing your anxiety. Kindness helps you feel more positive and better able to deal with anxiety-producing situations.

You may think that kindness is a fixed trait; you've either got it or you don't. Not so. Kindness is a skill that you can build with practice, like training your attention through meditation. In this section, you'll learn techniques to grow kindness toward yourself and others. Not only will these tools reduce your anxiety, but they'll also leave you feeling happier and more socially connected.

33. Compassion

Do you remember when you first heard about the immigrant children who were separated from their parents at the border? This type of news naturally evokes sympathy for their predicament. How did you feel when you saw photos of them detained in prison-like facilities? Most likely, you wanted them to be freed from those inhumane conditions. This is compassion, the observation of suffering accompanied by the heartfelt wish that the suffering be alleviated.

We live in a very "me"-focused culture in which it's easy to become overly self-involved. However, that self-involvement is the root of what makes you anxious. It's said that when you're young and naive, you're always worrying what other people are thinking about you. When you are older and wiser, you realize everyone was just thinking about themselves. With worry and defensiveness, you build up armor around your heart to protect yourself from the imagined slings and arrows of others, but in doing so, you cut yourself off from connecting with them. Self-protection ends up causing a well of loneliness.

When practicing compassion, you choose from a place of love rather than from a place of fear, from a place of connection rather than self-isolation. In doing so, you begin to connect to something beyond your own worries and, ironically, begin to alleviate those worries. As Shantideva said, all happiness and joy are the consequences of cherishing the well-being of others, while all problems are the consequences of cherishing yourself.[48]

Placing importance on cultivating positive emotions is a relatively new endeavor in psychology. Historically, psychologists focused on psychopathology—what goes wrong with our minds. Daniel Goleman's bestseller *Emotional Intelligence* drew focus to the importance of positive emotions in supporting our ability to be high-functioning members of society.[49] He describes how some people with a high IQ struggle in life, whereas others, who have a more modest IQ, succeed. As social animals, our ability to thrive is dependent on our ability to get along with others, to read social cues, and to react appropriately to those cues. Compassion is an essential part of our ability to bond with our loved ones, as well as to connect with people outside our immediate social networks. It's critical to your emotional intelligence.

However, practicing compassion can be off-putting, because it involves turning your attention toward the plight of others and the uncomfortable sadness that that stirs up. You might believe that purposefully focusing on heartache would impede happiness. However, with compassion, a sweetness emerges that tempers the heartache.

Chögyam Trungpa Rinpoche, one of the first teachers to bring Tibetan Buddhism to the West, described relating to the pain of compassion as a kind of sadness:

> When you awaken your heart, you find to your surprise that your heart is empty. If you really look, you won't find anything tangible and solid. If you search for the awakened heart, if you put your hand through your rib cage and feel for it, there's nothing there but tenderness. You feel sore and soft, and if you open your eyes to the rest of the world, you feel tremendous sadness. Sadness doesn't come from being mistreated. You don't feel sad because someone has insulted you or because you feel impoverished. Rather, the sadness is unconditioned. It occurs because your heart is completely open and exposed. There is no skin or tissue covering it; it is pure, raw meat. Even if a tiny mosquito lands on it, you feel so touched. Your experience is raw and tender and so personal.[50]

Compassion practice also gives you an opportunity to encounter challenging emotions in a controlled, meditative setting. You learn to feel these emotions without being overwhelmed by them. Your tendency to avoid discomfort drives your anxiety. This practice helps you understand that emotions are normal. You learn to turn toward them and be curious about them. You find that you can deal with them, even conflictive emotions like anger, fear, and sadness. Some misunderstand that in trying to reduce their anxiety, they're trying to dampen all of their emotions. Compassion practice helps you recognize the benefit of awakening to the pain of the world around you. That tender-hearted sensitivity is a gift, not a hindrance.

You may have been especially hungry for social engagement during the COVID pandemic. Relating compassionately toward others provides a sense of connection that your anxious mind so desperately desires.

Finally, compassion can motivate you into action. Rather than complacently ignoring the suffering of others or turning away from it because you fear it will cause you anxiety and discomfort, the pain evoked by authentic compassion helps you to get up off your butt and do something that might actually help alleviate suffering.

PRACTICE

Earlier I discussed my anxiety around being harassed for being gay. As a result, I developed the anxious habit of avoiding eye contact with strangers. To overcome this habit, I practiced looking at people I passed while silently wishing them well. This provided a straightforward yet effective way to practice kindness while, at the same time, reducing my anxiety around strangers.

Granted, in some contexts it may feel inappropriate to look directly at strangers. If so, you can feel friendly toward them in your heart without directly gazing at them. Adapt the practice to fit the context you are in. If you force a situation, the awkwardness may produce more anxiety and cause you to withdraw further. The purpose is to ignite an inner swell of positive emotions toward people you encounter.

34. Self-Compassion

When we think of compassion, we think almost entirely of compassion toward someone else. When we relate to ourselves, our bodies, and our abilities, it's more often with self-criticism. However, best-selling author and mindfulness teacher Jack Kornfield asserts that "If your compassion does not include yourself, it is incomplete."[51]

Self-compassion invites you to be kind toward yourself when you are going through difficulties. This self-directed compassion makes it easier to accept the fact that challenges and failures are a natural part of life. It invites you to be more forgiving toward yourself—instead of layering on more criticism—when things don't go as planned.

Social media is an unexpected source of anxiety. When you scroll through your feeds, you typically see the smooth-sailing lives of others and thereby think that you are alone in your misfortune. You forget that your friends' posts are cherry-picked to highlight life's sweetest moments: vacations, anniversaries, promotions, new homes, and adorable puppies and babies. People rarely post about spats with their partners, losing jobs, or being downed by a virus.

Then, when everyday challenges show up at your doorstep, you feel as if you are being unfairly singled out by the universe. The attitude of unfairness leads you to fight against the adversity. Without acceptance, you end up causing more aggravation. Compassion helps you to meet these hiccups with more grace. You choose to be sweet with yourself in these moments of pain, rather than exacerbating the pain with resistance and criticism.

Using your Observer Tool to shift to a more objective perspective can also lessen the pain that comes from adversities. With a broader view, you're able to remember that trials and tribulations happen for everyone. And in remembering that other people have their share of pain, you can choose to carry your portion of pain with courage rather than self-pity.

PRACTICE

Do some self-compassion letter writing. First, journal about a problem that tends to make you feel bad about yourself, such as a perceived flaw, a relationship problem, or a failure at work or school. Explore what emotions come up—shame, anger, sadness, fear.

Next, think of an imaginary friend who is unconditionally accepting and compassionate; someone who knows all your strengths and weaknesses, understands your life history, and is aware of your current circumstances. Write a letter to yourself from that imaginary friend's perspective. What would your friend say to encourage you to face your problem? What words would they use to convey compassion? How would your friend remind you that you are only human? When you're done writing, put the letter away for a few weeks and reread it later. You might save it to reread occasionally and allow yourself to be soothed and comforted.

35. Compassion Research

The research on compassion consistently shows that greater self-compassion is linked to decreased anxiety and depression.[52] The reduction in anxiety is due in part to the fact that self-compassionate people are less self-critical. However, self-compassion offers protection against anxiety and depression above and beyond the influence of self-criticism and negative affect.[53]

Self-compassionate people have a better perspective on their problems and are less likely to feel isolated by them. They experience less anxiety and self-consciousness when reflecting on their difficulties. And self-compassionate people are able to acknowledge how they have contributed to making the situation difficult without feeling overwhelmed by guilt or shame.[54]

Not surprisingly, people who experience more positive emotions live longer and healthier lives.[55] One study showed how compassion meditation can generate positive emotions to influence one's overall well-being. People in the study were randomly assigned to either a six-week compassion meditation group or a wait-list control group (the latter received the meditation training at the completion of the study).[56]

Researchers discovered that participants with good emotion regulation at the beginning of the study excelled at generating positive emotions during the compassion meditation. Further, their ability to generate positive emotions was associated with feeling socially connected. In a type of upward spiral, the more socially connected they felt, the better they became at regulating their emotions. The take-home message is that it is possible for you to generate positive emotions in ways that make you physically and emotionally healthier. And generating positive emotions is exactly what you'll practice in the upcoming compassion meditation.

PRACTICE

Start by setting a general intention to be kinder to yourself and others. Your intention is like a planned route on a roadmap that points you in the direction you want to go. You can also think of specific situations where you would benefit from being kinder and set specific intentions around those situations. For example, *I will be more patient with my husband when he forgets my name.*

36. Building Your Kindness Tool

Of course, everyone agrees that it is good to be kind. It's a much trickier proposition to overcome well-entrenched habits that are unkind. Shifting habits takes effort, whether they are behavioral habits like eating better or emotional habits like being kinder. You can build more kindness into your routine using the mindful tools in this book.

First, bring awareness to notice the types of situations that provoke you to be unkind. For example, it's hard to be kind when you are feeling challenged or attacked. You can start by using your Observer Tool to acknowledge when you're facing a difficult moment.

This is challenging.

This hurts.

As we've discussed, anxious people usually add to the difficulty by resisting it, struggling against it, or blaming someone for it. You can reduce the suffering associated with difficulties by accepting them.

Suffering is a part of life.

Everyone has ups and downs.

It's okay that I'm in the midst of this challenge.

Then you can use your power of choice to decide how you want to handle the difficult moment. To incorporate more kindness, invite it.

May I be kind to myself in this moment.

As you develop your Kindness Tool, you can expect that your old, unkind habits will resurface. Don't give up on your intention just because things don't change overnight. Think about how many years you have been responding to stressful situations in unkind ways. Change requires practice and patience. One of my teachers, Larry Yang, encouraged us to take a stepwise approach to being kinder. Ask yourself: *If I cannot be loving in this moment, can I be kind? If I cannot be kind, can I be nonjudgmental? If I cannot be nonjudgmental, can I not cause harm? And if I cannot not cause harm, can I cause the least harm possible?*

It's a lot to ask of yourself to suddenly be loving all the time. Setting the intention to be kinder is part of the practice. Start there. It may seem impossible to be loving toward someone who has hurt you or toward a group that you see doing harm in the world. Don't sugarcoat reality just to claim that you're compassionate. You first need to be mindfully honest about how you are feeling instead of taking a spiritual bypass from reality to achieve some idealized, saint-like state of being. Self-compassion includes honoring your truth. Author and civil rights activist Nikki Giovanni once said that being able to admit honestly that she didn't like white people was the first step in starting to like them.

Taking baby steps toward kindness allows you to release your expectation of suddenly becoming a saint. Since your anxious brain tends to highlight failure and skip over successes, be sure to congratulate yourself when you experience little wins practicing kindness.

PRACTICE

Moment of Kindness. Set a timer that alerts you at hourly intervals. When notified, pause whatever you are doing and ask, *How can I make this moment kinder?* Are there kind words that you can say? Is there some action that would boost kindness toward yourself or others? By purposefully peppering your day with kind moments, you will build kindness into a habit.

Inner and Outer Smile. Smiling is associated with kindness. You can jump-start kindness by putting a smile on your face. This can be an actual physical smile or a more subtle, inner smile. Try thinking of something sweet that helps activate your kindness. When I think of my dog, Sophie, my inner smile glows automatically. A forced smile can seem inauthentic, but even a forced smile leans your brain toward kindness. Further, a smiling face is contagious. Your smile will evoke smiles from people you pass, and in noticing their smiles, you'll feel happier and smile more. Like begets like.

Inner Smile Meditation. You can follow the guided meditation on the book's website (http://www.newharbinger.com/48817 —audio accessory 8: Inner Smile Meditation) or use the instructions below.

Find a comfortable position, either seated or lying down. Enhance the feeling of self-care by gently placing one hand on your heart and one hand on your belly. Feel the gentle pressure and warmth where your hands touch your torso. Feel free to experiment with other hand placements to find what feels best for you.

Take a deep breath in and, with a sighing exhale, let go of any tension that you're holding. Be especially aware of places where you know you carry stress. Take two more deep inhales followed by sighing exhales.

Now add a little smile, a slight upward curl of the corners of your mouth, or a slight twinkle in your eyes. Notice how changing your face affects how you feel. Imagine your heart with a smile, your belly. Feel the warmth of your smile infuse your whole being. Even your fingers and your toes smile. Let your attentional spotlight scan through your body and invite a smile into wherever your mind flows.

Nurturing Hand Gestures. Humans need physical attention. During the COVID pandemic, we grew starved of giving and receiving friendly physical touch like handshakes, hugs, and arm-in-arm walks. You can give yourself physical attention that both enhances your self-kindness and calms your nerves. For example, try placing one hand on your heart and the other on your belly. Take a moment to feel those points of connection and notice how holding your heart and belly make you feel. Can you add kind inner words to this moment? You can also experiment with a self-hug while gently rocking yourself or placing a hand on your cheek. Anything that feels nurturing will help. With these body gestures, you begin to cultivate a sweetness toward yourself that counters your habit of being harsh and self-critical.

In the context of this book, these compassion practices help to reduce your anxiety. However, I believe that as we make these changes in ourselves, our actions reverberate out into the world around us. Think globally, act locally. The act of creating a friendlier world starts right here, with you.

37. Compassion Meditation

Compassion meditation acts as a type of self-psychotherapy. It helps relieve difficult emotions, like fear and anger, by purposefully cultivating positive emotions, like kindness. It helps you develop a friendlier attitude toward yourself so that you are more self-accepting. Further, it improves your ability to regulate your emotional ups and downs and enhances your feelings of social connection.

You can follow the guided meditation on the book's website (http://www.newharbinger.com/48817—audio accessory 9: Self-Compassion Meditation) or use the instructions below.

First, find a comfortable position, either lying down or seated. Take a moment to settle your body by slowing your breath, and imagine releasing any tension into the earth as you exhale. If you become distracted or overwhelmed, come back to feeling your body resting and breathing right here.

Next, we'll go through five stages of developing compassion. If you want to create a shorter session, you can practice any of these stages on their own.

Stage 1. Bring to mind someone who cares about you—a friend or family member. It could be someone living or someone who has passed. Picture them looking at you with their warm eyes and loving smile. Open to the feeling of being cared for by them.

What does it feel like to be on the receiving end of that care? How does it feel in your heart...your face...or in other parts of your body? Without straining, can you open to this feeling of being cared about?

Sometimes, during this practice, you'll notice feelings other than kindness. This is expected and fine. When different feelings arise, like feeling ashamed or unworthy of care, accept those feelings. Then gently return your attention to feeling cared about by this loved one. Continue for a few minutes.

Now let go of your focus on this person, and thank them for their kindness and love.

Stage 2. Bring to mind someone whom you love. This could be a partner, a friend, a child, a parent, a coworker, a favorite aunt or uncle, or an animal friend. Sometimes our animal friends make the best partners for practicing compassion, because it's usually easy for us to feel that tenderness in our hearts when we think of them. This practice focuses on awaking your tender-heartedness. Use whoever helps you develop that feeling.

As you picture this person or animal friend, acknowledge that they face challenges and sometimes suffer. Accompany this acknowledgment by a heartfelt wish that they might suffer less.

As you consider their suffering, your mind might be thrown into worry or pulled back into your own pain. Your brain is adept at making associations, so it's natural for your mind to wander. When you notice that your mind has wandered, note to yourself, *Thinking,* to acknowledge the mind-wandering, and return to compassion.

Continue feeling compassion for with this person or animal for a few minutes. Then release your focus on them, thanking them for being in your life.

Stage 3. Bring to mind an image of yourself as a child, remembering a difficult time in your childhood when you were struggling, afraid, or angry. As you imagine the child, imagine your present, adult self sitting with your child self. You might imagine embracing the child or sitting with your arm around them—any gestures that relay comfort.

You might express compassion with kind thoughts silently spoken, *It is okay* or *It gets better,* or other words more specific to the challenges the child was facing, *It is not your fault.*

Like layers of an onion, these younger layers of your psyche are still present today. You now wish that those younger layers of yourself be held in compassion rather than criticism or shame.

Stage 4. Next, move forward in time through your childhood and continue to send compassion at important transitions in your life, especially reflecting on any difficult periods. Send compassion to yourself as you went through adolescence, as you left home and moved into your young adulthood.

Eventually, bring your awareness to your present self and continue to generate compassion. We all face challenges. Can you hold your present challenges kindly? Maybe add specific thoughts, like *May I forgive myself, May I accept my body and its continual changes,* or *May this pain pass away.* Find phrases that stir your heart.

Stage 5. To finish, release the focus on the self, and take a perspective shift. Imagine your awareness hovering in the sky above you. Look down on your town and recognize that many people in your town are facing difficulties. Some of them are homeless and hungry. Some are sick and in pain. Some of your neighbors are living with domestic violence and are afraid for their well-being. Some are lonely. Can you send out a wish that all the people in your town feel loved and accepted, and that all the people in your town find more ease and peace amid their challenges?

Finally, take your awareness even higher, so you can gaze down and see the whole planet. Send out these wishes: *May all beings feel safe. May all beings be as healthy as they can be at this moment. May all beings find peace.*

Next, draw your awareness back down to feel yourself resting right here. Feel your connection to the earth. Feel your breath flowing gently in and out.

Notice how you feel at the end of the practice. Allow yourself the space to rest in this state of compassion and ease for a while longer.

When you're ready to conclude, thank yourself for taking this time to practice. Building kindness toward yourself and others is a step toward creating greater peace for us all.

SUMMARY OF THE KINDNESS TOOL

You tend to see your anxiety as a personal flaw and are there-fore judgmental and ashamed about it. But judgment and shame only make your anxiety worse. One proven remedy is to be kind to yourself when things are difficult, rather than blaming yourself for not measuring up. Kindness soothes the anxious mind and makes whatever you're facing easier to manage. Remember that it's not the people and events in your life that make you anxious. Instead, it's your reactions to those people and events. The outer landscape is less important than the inner attitude. So when you create an inner attitude of kindness, you naturally turn off the anxiety and start to feel more at ease with yourself and the world.

Understanding
Rest and Digest

Throughout this book I've discussed the fight-or-flight response, the automatic physiological response that ramps up your metabolism to help you deal with threats. In this last chapter, I want to tell you about its complementary system, called the "rest and digest response." It's the yin to the fight-or-flight's yang. Rest and digest is an automatic, unconscious response that puts the brakes on fight-or-flight activity to help you calm down after an upset.

If the brakes aren't working well, the fight-or-flight system isn't properly suppressed, and you remain anxiously aroused even after the stress-inducing event has passed. You also get stuck ruminating on your problems instead of bouncing back from them.

38. The Vagus Nerve and Anxiety

The vagus nerve is the central player in your rest and digest system and is critical to managing your anxiety. It is the largest and perhaps most important nerve in your whole body. I know it's hard to get excited about physiology. But, even if you are only "vagally" interested, keep reading.

The word "vagus" means "wandering" in Latin, which is an appropriate moniker for a nerve that wanders from the base of the brain all the way to the colon, with numerous whistle stops along the way. Information runs in two directions on the vagus highway. It can relay information from your body to your brain and can also send messages from the brain back down to control your body.

The vagus nerve modifies your arousal, respiration, heart rate, and attention in response to stress. One of the most crucial roles of the vagus nerve is controlling your heart rate. When you are anxious, your heart rate and blood pressure go up. The vagus nerve slows the heart rate and lowers your blood pressure to help you settle after an upset.

"Vagal tone" refers to the activity of the vagus nerve and reflects a measure of your body's ability to handle stress. When your vagal tone is low, the vagus nerve isn't calming your body effectively. Low vagal tone is like having low brake fluid in your car; your brakes still work, but not very well. Researchers have discovered that by increasing your vagal tone, you can enhance both mental and physical well-being. High vagal tone reflects a healthy rest and digest system and is associated with many markers of good mental health:

- your ability to regulate your emotions[57]

- your capacity to cope with stress[58]

- your inclination to be more socially engaged[59]

- your tendency to be concerned for the well-being of others[60]

- your tendency to act with kindness toward others[61]

- your feelings of warmth when you witness altruistic actions[62]

- your experience of compassion when you witness human suffering[63]

Sounds great, right? Well, let's first take a look at how to measure vagal tone.

39. Measuring Vagal Tone

Vagal tone is typically based on your heart rate variability (HRV). Some smart watches are now capable of monitoring HRV to track stress continuously throughout the day and to display stress scores that indicate when you're having a stress reaction. The watch can detect stress before you even realize that you're anxious, because it is measuring one of the earliest indicators of stress (changes in your HRV) to let you know that your fight-or-flight system has been triggered. Yay, technology.

So, what is this HRV that the smart watch is measuring? In healthy people, heart rate is coupled to the breath cycle; your heart rate increases when you inhale and decreases when you exhale. You can actually feel this yourself—you don't need a smart watch.

PRACTICE

First, use your right middle finger to find your pulse on your left wrist. Once you have found it, close your eyes and inhale for six heart beats, and exhale for six heart beats. Continue for about a minute.

You'll notice that your heart rate speeds up slightly as you breathe in and slows down as you breathe out. This normal fluctuation in the heart's rhythm is referred to as "respiratory sinus arrhythmia," a measure of HRV.

As an aside, you can use heart-synchronized breathing to bolster the calming effects of your rest and digest system. For example, try using your heartbeat to keep time for you as you practice Relaxation Breathing. Inhale for three heartbeats, exhale for six heartbeats, and then pause for three heartbeats. Try this for one minute and notice how you feel.

So HRV is an indicator of your vagal tone, which reflects how well your rest and digest system is functioning. Let's now look at how HRV relates to anxiety.

40. Heart Rate Variability and Anxiety

Since the vagus nerve is the main nerve of your rest-and-digest system, HRV provides a window into seeing how well the overall rest and digest system is working.[64] Though it may seem farfetched, scientists propose that your heart rate provides one of the best indicators of your ability to regulate your emotions.[65] Why?

Interestingly, the frontal lobe structures involved in emotion regulation are mostly the same ones involved in cardiac control.[66] The common denominator between your heart rate and your emotions is your frontal brain. People with poor frontal lobe function have low HRV, are more anxious, and show poor emotional control.

People with anxiety disorders have disrupted HRV,[67] and the severity of the disruption relates to their clinical ratings of how anxious they are.[68] Thus HRV has been used to predict how well patients will respond to therapy.[69] The HRV pattern in patients with anxiety shows that their fight-or-flight system gets turned on and then stays on, even when circumstances don't warrant it. They have the gas pedal that ramps up their anxious arousal, but insufficient braking power to calm themselves back down.

You've undoubtedly noticed times when you felt on edge and agitated or had a hard time sitting still or sleeping, even when nothing was amiss at the moment. This may reflect your fight-or-flight system getting stuck on high, and your rest and digest response not doing its job of calming you. This doesn't necessarily mean you have clinical levels of anxiety. HRV has been shown to get disrupted in people suffering from everyday stressors. For example, college students show a lowered HRV the night before a big exam. Further, their night-before HRV predicts how anxious they will feel at exam time.[70]

Interestingly, your current HRV can forecast how anxious you'll likely be in the future. For instance, in one longitudinal study of nearly a thousand adolescents, lower HRV scores at the beginning of the study predicted their anxiety scores a full two years later.[71]

Developmentally, the relationship between HRV and anxiety is set up early in life; low HRV relates to social anxiety in preschoolers.[72] Further, newborns mimic the vagal tone of their mothers. Anxious moms who have low HRV during their pregnancy have newborns with low vagal tone.[73] But despite how it may seem, given its early onset, HRV is not a fixed trait. In the next chapter, I'll describe how you can increase your HRV to enhance your vagal tone and improve your capacity to calm yourself down.

But before I jump into that, let me add one more dot to the connection between anxiety and the inability to calm the fight-or-flight cycle—inhibition. Inhibition is an important function of the frontal lobes, and there are many examples of poor inhibition contributing to anxiety. When upsets occur, people who are anxious are less able to constrain their knee-jerk responses. The automatic reactions coming from your fear brain are about survival and rarely reflect your most tactful responses. For example, imagine if your boss berated you in front of your coworkers. Your primal defense might be to hurl back some snarky response, but your wiser frontal brain could reason that yelling at your boss is not a great strategy for job longevity and thus suppress your sarcasm. With more time to think, you may even be able to generate compassion toward your boss, recognizing that they were probably yelling at you because they're also under a lot of pressure. Overall, being able to inhibit automatic reactions allows you to navigate difficult interactions with more finesse. Having less flexibility in responding can exacerbate your feelings of lack of control and fuel your anxiety, not to mention get you into a heap of trouble when you blurt out something that you'll later regret.

The good news is that you can improve your ability to inhibit automatic reactions, so you don't spew the first angry words that pop into your mind or automatically get swept away into a storm of anxious catastrophizing.

Training your attention is a central part of every mindfulness meditation. As such, all of the mindful practices in this book serve to enhance frontal lobe control. Just like regular trips to the gym help keep your muscles toned, regular meditation helps keep your frontal lobes performing at their peak. For example, one skill you practice during meditation is inhibiting the intrusive thoughts that distract you from your breath or body. The more you practice switching your attentional spotlight back to where you want it to be, the stronger your attentional system will become. With practice, you will get better at switching away from automatic, fear-based reactions that your amygdala spews out.

41. Increasing Your Vagal Tone

If your vagal tone is low, don't worry. You can increase it by practicing some of these research-proven techniques already in your toolbox.

- controlled, deep belly breathing

- singing or humming (the Bee's Breath)

- mindfulness meditations (like the Body Scan or Walking Meditation)

- self-massage

- compassion meditation

- cold exposure—this technique isn't covered in this book; researchers have found that exposing your body to short bouts of cold (taking a cold shower, going out in cold temperatures without warm clothes) activates your vagus nerve to increase vagal tone

To improve and maintain high vagal tone, it's helpful to integrate these techniques into your daily routine. For example, instead of jumping out of bed at the sound of your alarm, pause and take ten deep belly breaths before you get up. If taking a cold shower sounds too off-putting, try just one minute of cold water at the end of your warm shower or simply splash your face with cold water at the sink. Find a time during the day for a regular meditation practice, like a Body Scan or compassion meditation. Take a pause during your day for a five-minute Grounding Self-Massage. Walk to and from your car mindfully. I'm sure you can think of many other ways of creating little mindful moments in your day, like brushing your teeth or drinking your coffee mindfully.

With just a little effort, you will soon reap the calming benefits of these practices. With improved vagal tone, both the frequency and intensity of your anxiety will decrease. You will feel more grounded and better able to regulate your emotions. You will feel less driven by fear-based impulses and thus able to make wiser choices. You will feel more socially connected. Most importantly, you will develop a sense of trust in your own ability to improve your mental and emotional well-being.

SUMMARY OF YOUR
REST AND DIGEST SYSTEM

Anxiety flourishes when your rest and digest system isn't working well. The frontal lobes have insufficient braking power to calm down your fight-or-flight arousal. Therefore, you get stuck in anxious arousal even when no immediate threats are present. This deficiency is expressed as low vagal tone and is usually measured by HRV.

With poor frontal lobe control, the more rudimentary fear centers of your brain drive what you think, say, and do. You react impulsively instead of responding mindfully.

Luckily, your frontal lobes can be trained to improve response inhibition and increase your vagal tone. Many of the practices in this book involve increasing your ability to pay attention, which will help tune up your frontal lobes and enhance your response inhibition. With practice, you become more able to notice fear-based thoughts without getting stuck in them and to recognize fear-based impulses without acting on them. When you're not being driven by fear, you can choose from something other than fear. As Ambrose Redmoon writes, "Courage is not the absence of fear, but rather the judgment that something else is more important than fear."[74]

Conclusion

Let me boil down the essence of this book into its most important take-home points. First, anxiety is a natural part of life. Through human evolution, we all have inherited anxious brains. Trying to suppress your anxiety only makes it worse. So the goal in this approach is not to eliminate anxiety, but to change your relationship to it. You learn to acknowledge it and cope with it so that it doesn't interfere with your performance and sense of well-being.

The first step involves becoming aware of when anxious symptoms arise. It makes logical sense that you have to notice symptoms before you can do anything about them. Otherwise, they continue to wreak havoc under the radar of your awareness. Once you have become aware of an anxious symptom, you accept it. Your mind may want to resist, avoid, or control your anxious symptoms. But when you struggle against them, they bother you more. When you accept them, they bother you less.

The Breathing and Grounding Tools help you to quiet your flight-or-flight response, so you feel more at ease. When you're not driven by anxiety, it's easier to make skillful choices that aren't based in fear. The Kindness Tool helps you relate to yourself in a friendlier way. Instead of entrenching your anxiety with self-criticism and shame, you choose to be kind by allowing yourself to be as you are.

Understanding these tools is not complicated. However, putting them into practice can be challenging, mostly because it involves overcoming all of the fear-based habits that you have been rehearsing for years, like worrying, catastrophizing, and self-criticizing.

Speaking for myself and my students, the hardest part of mindfulness is remembering to use it. That said, I encourage you to think of ways that you can remind yourself to use your tools. For example, you can put your daily meditation in your calendar, just as you would a meeting or an appointment. You can place sticky notes on your bathroom mirror or fridge reminding yourself: *Just breathe.* Or on the dashboard of your car: *Just drive.* You can set an alarm on your computer to remind yourself to stand up occasionally to take a Peaceful Pause. You can make a regular date with a friend or family member to mindfully walk together. Knowing about these tools is not enough. They only work their magic when you use them.

And when you do use them, you will notice the payoff. By being more accepting of your experience of anxiety, you can drop the struggle against it and live a more grounded and peaceful life. And as you become more peaceful, you create little ripples of peace that touch those around you. Desmond Tutu said, "Do your little bit of good where you are; it's those little bits of good put together that overwhelm the world."

I wish you the very best as you continue to put these mindful tools to work. Be patient. Practice the meditations. Reread chapters when you need a refresher. Keep breathing. You *can* change your relationship to anxiety. In fact, you already have.

Sharing Your Experience

If you made it this far in the book, congratulations. I appreciate your willingness to explore these practices. My intention is to help people like you alleviate their anxiety by using these mindful tools. You can support that intention by sharing what you've learned with people you know. Teach a friend who's struggling how to breathe deeply or guide a child in a Five-Senses Grounding Meditation. Tell your anxious friends about this book or share your experience with a wider audience. Through your encouragement, you can help others reduce their suffering.

Acknowledgments

I have been blessed with so many wonderful teachers throughout my lifetime. I would especially like to thank a few who have shared from their wells of knowledge in each of their respective fields.

Yoga: Janet Stone, Annie Carpenter, Richard Rosen, and David Goulet.

Mindfulness: Jon Kabat-Zinn, Jack Kornfield, and Larry Yang.

Psychology and Neuroscience: Lyn Raible, Herbert Pick, Chuck Nelson, and Yaakov Stern.

Anatomy and Massage: Brian Bucchiarelli, Therdchai Chumphoopong (Mac), and Stacy Kinirons.

I offer my deep appreciation to my husband, Steven, whose constant encouragement has supported me in exploring the path of mindful healing. Thank you for your word-bird editing skills that helped make this book more user-friendly. Thank you for your unending love and support. You are my favorite anxiolytic.

Finally, I want to thank the staff at New Harbinger for their guidance and assistance in helping bring these ideas to you.

Endnotes

1   W. James, *The Principles of Psychology* (New York: H. Holt, 1890).

2   Ibid.

3   A. Nin, *Seduction of the Minotaur* (London: Penguin, 1993).

4   Y. Masaoka and I. Homma, "Anxiety and Respiratory Patterns: Their Relationship During Mental Stress and Physical Load," *International Journal of Psychophysiology* 27, no. 2 (1997): 153–59.

5   J. L. Herrero et al., "Breathing Above the Brain Stem: Volitional Control and Attentional Modulation in Humans," *Journal of Neurophysiology* 119, no. 1 (2018) 145–59.

6   G. P. Chrousos, "Stress and Disorders of the Stress System," *Nature Reviews: Endocrinology* 5, no. 5 (2009): 374–81.

7   E.-J. Kim and J. E. Dimsdale, "The Effect of Psychosocial Stress on Sleep: A Review of Polysomnographic Evidence," *Behavioral Sleep Medicine* 5, no. 4 (2007): 256–78.

8   B. S. McEwen, "Protection and Damage from Acute and Chronic Stress: Allostasis and Allostatic Overload and Relevance to the Pathophysiology of Psychiatric Disorders," *Annals of the New York Academy of Sciences* 1032, no. 1 (2004): 1–7.

9   S. C. Segerstrom and G. E. Miller, "Psychological Stress and the Human Immune System: A Meta-Analytic Study of Thirty Years of Inquiry," *Psychological Bulletin* 130, no. 4 (2004): 601–30.

10   R. A. Fabes and N. Eisenberg, "Regulatory Control and
     Adults' Stress-Related Responses to Daily Life Events," *Journal
     of Personality and Social Psychology* 73, no. 5 (1997): 1107–17; R.
     P. Nolan et al., "Heart Rate Variability Biofeedback as a
     Behavioral Neurocardiac Intervention to Enhance Vagal Heart
     Rate Control," *American Heart Journal* 149, no. 6 (2005): 1137;
     R. Gevirtz, The Promise of Heart Rate Variability
     Biofeedback: Evidence-Based Applications," *Biofeedback* 41, no.
     3 (2013): 110–20; and I. Dziembowska et al., "Effects of Heart
     Rate Variability Biofeedback on EEG Alpha Asymmetry and
     Anxiety Symptoms in Male Athletes: A Pilot Study," *Applied
     Psychophysiology and Biofeedback* 41, no. 2 (2016): 141–50.

11   G. J. Asmundson and M. B. Stein, "Vagal Attenuation in Panic
     Disorder: An Assessment of Parasympathetic Nervous System
     Function and Subjective Reactivity to Respiratory Manipulations,"
     Psychosomatic Medicine 56, no. 3 (1994): 187–93; R. M. Kaushik et
     al., "Effects of Mental Relaxation and Slow Breathing in Essential
     Hypertension," *Complementary Therapies in Medicine* 14, no. 2
     (2006): 120–26; R. P. Brown and P. L. Gerbarg, "Sudarshan Kriya
     Yogic Breathing in the Treatment of Stress, Anxiety, and
     Depression. Part II—Clinical Applications and Guidelines,"
     Journal of Alternative and Complementary Medicine 11, no. 4 (2005):
     711–17.

12   M. A. Katzman et al., "A Multicomponent Yoga-Based, Breath
     Intervention Program as an Adjunctive Treatment in Patients
     Suffering from Generalized Anxiety Disorder with or without
     Comorbidities," *International Journal of Yoga* 5, no. 1 (2012): 57–65.

13   E. M. Seppälä et al., "Breathing-Based Meditation Decreases
     Posttraumatic Stress Disorder Symptoms in US Military Veterans:
     A Randomized Controlled Longitudinal Study," *Journal of
     Traumatic Stress* 27, no. 4 (2014): 397–405.

14 O. L. Carter et al., "Meditation Alters Perceptual Rivalry in Tibetan Buddhist Monks," *Current Biology* 15, no. 11 (2005): R412–13.

15 B. K. Hölzel et al., "Mindfulness Practice Leads to Increases in Regional Brain Gray Matter Density," *Psychiatry Research* 191, no. 1 (2011) 36–43; A. Doll et al., "Mindful Attention to Breath Regulates Emotions via Increased Amygdala-Prefrontal Cortex Connectivity," *Neuroimage* 134 (2016): 305–13; and W. Kersemaekers et al., "A Workplace Mindfulness Intervention May Be Associated with Improved Psychological Well-Being and Productivity: A Preliminary Field Study in a Company Setting," *Frontiers in Psychology* 9 (2018): 195.

16 M. Ghaly and D. Teplitz, "The Biologic Effects of Grounding the Human Body During Sleep as Measured by Cortisol Levels and Subjective Reporting of Sleep, Pain, and Stress," *Journal of Alternative and Complementary Medicine* 10, no. 5 (2004): 767–76; D. Brown, G. Chevalier, and M. Hill, "Pilot Study on the Effect of Grounding on Delayed-Onset Muscle Soreness," *Journal of Alternative and Complementary Medicine* 16, no. 3 (2010): 265–73; and J. L. Oschman, G. Chevalier, and R. Brown, "The Effects of Grounding (Earthing) on Inflammation, the Immune Response, Wound Healing, and Prevention and Treatment of Chronic Inflammatory and Autoimmune Diseases," *Journal of Inflammation Research* 8 (2015): 83–96.

17 W. J. Nichols, *Blue Mind: The Surprising Science That Shows How Being near, in, on, or under Water Can Make You Happier, Healthier, More Connected and Better at What You Do* (New York: Little, Brown, 2014).

18 A. Kjellgren and J. Westman, "Beneficial Effects of Treatment with Sensory Isolation in Flotation-Tank as a Preventive Health-Care Intervention: A Randomized Controlled Pilot Trial," *BMC Complementary and Alternative Medicine* 14, no. 1 (2014): 417.

19   C. I. Seresinhe et al., "Happiness Is Greater in More Scenic Locations," *Scientific Reports* 9, no. 1 (2019): 4498.

20   G. Mackerron and S. Mourato, "Happiness Is Greater in Natural Environments," *Global Environmental Change* 23 (2013): 992–1000; and C. A. Capaldi, R. L. Dopko, and J. M. Zelenski, "The Relationship Between Nature Connectedness and Happiness: A Meta-Analysis," *Frontiers in Psychology* 5 (2014): 976.

21   E. K. Nisbet and J. M. Zelenski, "The NR-6: A New Brief Measure of Nature Relatedness," *Frontiers in Psychology* 4 (2013): 813.

22   J. Barton and M. Rogerson, "The Importance of Greenspace for Mental Health," *BJPsych International* 14, no. 4 (2017): 79–81.

23   Q. Li, "Effect of Forest Bathing Trips on Human Immune Function," *Environmental Health and Preventive Medicine* 15, no. 1 (2010): 9–17.

24   G. Chevalier et al., "Earthing: Health Implications of Reconnecting the Human Body to the Earth's Surface Electrons," *Journal of Environmental and Public Health* 2012 (2012): 2915411.

25   D, Hunt, "Peace Is This Moment Without Judgment," in *Leaves from Moon Mountain: Poems and Reflections* (San Francisco: Moon Mountain Sangha Publishing, 2015), 132.

26   Epictetus, *Enchiridion,* trans. George Long (Mineola, NY: Dover, 2004).

27   J. Patel and P. Patel, "Consequences of Repression of Emotion: Physical Health, Mental Health and General Well Being," *International Journal of Psychotherapy Practice and Research* 1 (2019) 16–21.

28   V. Ramseyer Winter et al., "Body Appreciation, Anxiety, and Depression Among a Racially Diverse Sample of Women," *Journal of Health Psychology* 24, no. 11 (2019): 1517–25.

29 R. McCraty et al. "The Impact of a New Emotional Self-Management Program on Stress, Emotions, Heart Rate Variability, DHEA and Cortisol," *Integrative Physiological and Behavioral Science* 33, no. 2 (1998): 151–70.

30 Y. J. Wong et al., "Does Gratitude Writing Improve the Mental Health of Psychotherapy Clients? Evidence from a Randomized Controlled Trial," *Psychotherapy Research* 28, no. 2 (2018): 192–202.

31 P. Kini et al., "The Effects of Gratitude Expression on Neural Activity," *Neuroimage* 128 (2016): 1–10.

32 W. James, *The Principles of Psychology* (New York: H. Holt, 1890).

33 V. E. Frankl, *Man's Search for Meaning* (Boston: Beacon Press, 2006).

34 M. Maltz, *Psycho-Cybernetics* (New York: Simon and Schuster, 1993).

35 P. Lally et al., "How Are Habits Formed: Modelling Habit Formation in the Real World," *European Journal of Social Psychology* 40, no. 6 (2010): 998–1009.

36 W. Wood and D. T. Neal, "A New Look at Habits and the Habit-Goal Interface," *Psychological Review* 114, no. 4 (2007): 843–63.

37 Ibid.

38 W. Wood, J. M. Quinn, and D. A. Kashy, "Habits in Everyday Life: Thought, Emotion, and Action," *Journal of Personality and Social Psychology* 83, no. 6 (2002): 1281–97.

39 T. D. Barnes et al., "Activity of Striatal Neurons Reflects Dynamic Encoding and Recoding of Procedural Memories," *Nature* 437, no. 7062 (2005): 1158–61.

40 M. Williamson, *A Return to Love: Reflections on the Principles of "A Course in Miracles"* (New York: HarperOne, 1996).

41 Dass, R., *Be Here Now* (San Cristobal, NM: Lama Foundation, 1971).

42 M. A. Killingsworth and D. T. Gilbert, "A Wandering Mind Is an Unhappy Mind," *Science* 330, no. 6006 (2010): 932.

43 J. P. Jamieson et al. "Turning the Knots in Your Stomach into Bows: Reappraising Arousal Improves Performance on the GRE," *Journal of Experimental Social Psychology* 46, no. 1 (2009): 208–212.

44 R. E. Emery and L. Laumann-Billings, "An Overview of the Nature, Causes, and Consequences of Abusive Family Relationships: Toward Differentiating Maltreatment and Violence," *American Psychologist* 53, no. 2 (1998): 121–35; J. M. Golding, "Intimate Partner Violence as a Risk Factor for Mental Disorders: A Meta-Analysis," *Journal of Family Violence* 14, no. 2 (1999): 99–132; and V. J. Edwards et al., "Relationship Between Multiple Forms of Childhood Maltreatment and Adult Mental Health in Community Respondents: Results from the Adverse Childhood Experiences Study," *American Journal of Psychiatry* 160, no. 8 (2003): 1453–60.

45 M. D. Seery, E. A. Holman, and R. C. Silver, "Whatever Does Not Kill Us: Cumulative Lifetime Adversity, Vulnerability, and Resilience," *Journal of Personality and Social Psychology* 99, no. 6 (2010): 1025–41.

46 R. A. Dienstbier, "Arousal and Physiological Toughness: Implications for Mental and Physical Health. *Psychological Review* 96, no. 1 (1989): 84–100.

47 R. Harris, *The Happiness Trap: How to Stop Struggling and Start Living* (Boston: Shambhala; Wollombi, Australia: Exisle, 2007).

48 Shantideva, *The Way of the Bodhisattva* (Boston: Shambhala, 2006).

49 Daniel Goleman, Emotional *Intelligence: Why It Can Matter More than IQ* (New York: Bantam, 2005).

50 Chögyam Trungpa, C.R.G., *Shambhala: The Sacred Path of the Warrior* (Boston: Shambhala, 2007).

51 J. Kornfield, *Buddha's Little Instruction Book* (New York: Bantam, 1994).

52 A. MacBeth and A. Gumley, "Exploring Compassion: A Meta-Analysis of the Association Between Self-Compassion and Psychopathology," *Clinical Psychology Review* 32, no. 6 (2012): 545–52.

53 R. Warren, E. Smeets, and K. Neff, "Being Compassionate to Oneself Is Associated with Emotional Resilience and Psychological Well-Being," *Current Psychiatry* 15, no. 12 (2016): 19–33.

54 M. R. Leary et al., "Self-Compassion and Reactions to Unpleasant Self-Relevant Events: The Implications of Treating Oneself Kindly," *Journal of Personality and Social Psychology* 92, no. 5 (2007): 887–904.

55 R. T. Howell, M. L. Kern, and S. Lyubomirsky, "Health Benefits: Meta-Analytically Determining the Impact of Well-Being on Objective Health Outcomes," *Health Psychology Review* 1, no. 1 (2007): 83–136.

56 B. E. Kok et al., "How Positive Emotions Build Physical Health: Perceived Positive Social Connections Account for the Upward Spiral Between Positive Emotions and Vagal Tone," *Psychological Science* 24, no. 7 (2013): 1123–32.

57 J. F. Thayer et al., "Heart Rate Variability, Prefrontal Neural Function, and Cognitive Performance: The Neurovisceral Integration Perspective on Self-Regulation, Adaptation, and Health," *Annals of Behavioral Medicine* 37, no. 2 (2009): 141–53.

58 R. A. Fabes and N. Eisenberg, "Regulatory Control and Adults' Stress-Related Responses to Daily Life Events," *Journal of Personality and Social Psychology* 73, no. 5 (1997): 1107–17.

59 M. Horsten et al., "Psychosocial Factors and Heart Rate
    Variability in Healthy Women," *Psychosomatic Medicine*
    61, no. 1 (1999): 49–57.

60 B. Bornemann et al., "Helping from the Heart: Voluntary
    Upregulation of Heart Rate Variability Predicts Altruistic
    Behavior," *Biological Psychology* 119 (2016): 54–63.

61 B. E. Kok et al., "How Positive Emotions Build Physical Health:
    Perceived Positive Social Connections Account for the Upward
    Spiral Between Positive Emotions and Vagal Tone," *Psychological
    Science* 24, no. 7 (2013): 1123–32.

62 J. S. Hutchinson, *The Heart of Elevation: Investigating the
    Physiological and Neural Mechanisms Underlying Moral Elevation*
    (honors college thesis, Oregon State University, 2012).

63 J. E. Stellar et al., "Affective and Physiological Responses to the
    Suffering of Others: Compassion and Vagal Activity," *Journal of
    Personality and Social Psychology* 108, no. 4, (2015): 572–85.

64 A. Sgoifo et al., "The Inevitable Link Between Heart and
    Behavior: New Insights from Biomedical Research and
    Implications for Clinical Practice," *Neuroscience and Biobehavioral
    Review* 33, no. 2 (2009): 61–62; and S. Laborde, E. Mosley, and
    A. Mertgen, "Vagal Tank Theory: The Three Rs of Cardiac Vagal
    Control Functioning—Resting, Reactivity, and Recovery,"
    Frontiers in Neuroscience 12 (2018): 458.

65 S. W. Porges, "The Polyvagal Perspective," *Biological Psychology,*
    74, no. 2 (2007): 116–43.

66 F. Beissner et al., "The Autonomic Brain: An Activation
    Likelihood Estimation Meta-Analysis for Central Processing of
    Autonomic Function," *Journal of Neuroscience* 33, no. 25 (2013):
    10503–11.

67   J. F. Thayer et al., "Phasic Heart Period Reactions to Cued Threat and Nonthreat Stimuli in Generalized Anxiety Disorder," *Psychophysiology* 37, no. 3 (2000): 361–68.

68   E. Klein et al., "Altered Heart Rate Variability in Panic Disorder Patients," *Biological Psychiatry* 37, no. 1 (1995): 18–24.

69   K. J. Mathewson et al., "Does Respiratory Sinus Arrhythmia (RSA) Predict Anxiety Reduction During Cognitive Behavioral Therapy (CBT) for Social Anxiety Disorder (SAD)?" *International Journal of Psychophysiology* 88, no. 2 (2013): 171–81.

70   M. Sakakibara et al., "Impact of Real-World Stress on Cardiorespiratory Resting Function During Sleep in Daily Life," *Psychophysiology* 45, no. 4 (2008): 667–70.

71   K. Greaves-Lord et al., "Reduced Autonomic Flexibility as a Predictor for Future Anxiety in Girls from the General Population: The TRAILS Study," *Psychiatry Research* 179, no. 2 (2010): 187–93.

72   P. D. Hastings et al., "Parental Socialization, Vagal Regulation, and Preschoolers' Anxious Difficulties: Direct Mothers and Moderated Fathers," *Child Development* 79, no. 1 (2008) 45–64.

73   N. A. Jones et al., "Newborns of Mothers with Depressive Symptoms Are Physiologically Less Developed," *Infant Behavior and Development* 21, no. 3 (1998): 537–41.

74   Ambrose Redmoon, "No Peaceful Warriors!" in *Gnosis: A Journal of the Western Inner Traditions,* vol. 21, *Holy War,* ed. by Jim Kinney (San Francisco: Lumen Foundation, Fall 1991), 40.

Domonick Wegesin, PhD, conducted cognitive neuroscience research on the aging brain as a professor of neuropsychology in Columbia University's department of neurology. He transitioned from academics into mind-body medicine, studying mindfulness-based stress reduction (MBSR) with Jon Kabat-Zinn and other senior teachers at the University of Massachusetts Medical Center. He currently teaches anxiety-reduction yoga classes and workshops in California.

ABOUT US

Founded by psychologist Matthew McKay and Patrick Fanning, New Harbinger has published books that promote wellness in mind, body, and spirit for more than forty-five years.

Our proven-effective self-help books and pioneering workbooks help readers of all ages and backgrounds make positive lifestyle changes, improve mental health and well-being, and achieve meaningful personal growth. In addition, our spirituality books offer profound guidance for deepening awareness and cultivating healing, self-discovery, and fulfillment.

New Harbinger is proud to be an independent and employee-owned company, publishing books that reflect its core values of integrity, innovation, commitment, sustainability, compassion, and trust. Written by leaders in the field and recommended by therapists worldwide, New Harbinger books are practical, reliable, and provide real tools for real change.

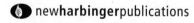 **newharbinger**publications

MORE BOOKS from
NEW HARBINGER PUBLICATIONS

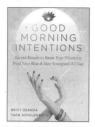
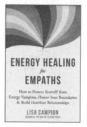
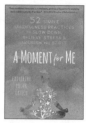
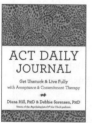
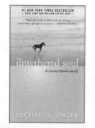
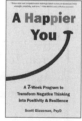

Did you know there are free tools you can download for this book?

Free tools are things like **worksheets, guided meditation exercises**, and **more** that will help you get the most out of your book.

You can download free tools for this book—whether you bought or borrowed it, in any format, from any source— from the **New Harbinger** website. All you need is a NewHarbinger.com account. Just use the URL provided in this book to view the free tools that are available for it. Then, click on the "download" button for the free tool you want, and follow the prompts that appear to log in to your NewHarbinger.com account and download the material.

You can also save the free tools for this book to your **Free Tools Library** so you can access them again anytime, just by logging in to your account! Just look for this button on the book's free tools page:

+ save this to my
free tools library

If you need help accessing or downloading free tools, visit **newharbinger.com/faq** or contact us at customerservice@newharbinger.com.

CELEBRATING
40 YEARS